MORTAL SECRETS

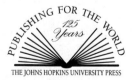

PUBLISHING FOR THE WORLD
125 Years
THE JOHNS HOPKINS UNIVERSITY PRESS

MORTAL SECRETS

TRUTH AND LIES IN THE AGE OF AIDS

ROBERT KLITZMAN, M.D.

Department of Psychiatry, College of Physicians and Surgeons, and Department of Sociomedical Sciences, Mailman School of Public Health, Columbia University, New York

and

RONALD BAYER, PH.D.

Department of Sociomedical Sciences, Mailman School of Public Health, Columbia University, New York

The Johns Hopkins University Press | *Baltimore and London*

© 2003 The Johns Hopkins University Press
All rights reserved. Published 2003
Printed in the United States of America on acid-free paper
9 8 7 6 5 4 3 2 1

The Johns Hopkins University Press
2715 North Charles Street
Baltimore, Maryland 21218-4363
www.press.jhu.edu

Library of Congress Cataloging-in-Publication Data
Klitzman, Robert.
    Mortal secrets: truth and lies in the age of AIDS /
Robert Klitzman and Ronald Bayer.
        p. cm.
Includes bibliographical references and index.
    ISBN 0-8018-7427-0 (acid-free)
    1. AIDS (Disease)—Prevention—Social aspects. 2. Self-
disclosure. 3. HIV-positive persons—Sexual behavior.
I. Bayer, Ronald. II. Title.
RA643.8.K56 2003
362.1'969792—dc21   2002156771

A catalog record for this book is available from the British
Library.

The opposite of the truth has
one hundred thousand faces,
and an infinite field

—MONTAIGNE

Tell all the truth
But tell it slant,
Success in circuit lies.

—EMILY DICKINSON

CONTENTS

ACKNOWLEDGMENTS

THIS BOOK could not have been written without the gracious assistance of many individuals. First and foremost, we wish to thank the men and women whom we interviewed—who shared with us their deepest secrets, pain, shame, and hopes. Without their candor and trust, this project would not have been possible.

We are deeply indebted to several funders. The National Institute of Mental Health provided a Mentored Clinical Scientist Career Development Award to one of us (RK) and a Research Scientist Award to the other (RB). It also supported the Ethics and Policy Core of the NIMH-funded HIV Center for Clinical and Behavioral Studies at the New York State Psychiatric Institute / Columbia University Department of Psychiatry, with which we are both affiliated. We also received valuable support through an Aaron Diamond Foundation Post-Doctoral Research Fellowship, a Russell Sage Foundation Visiting Scholar Award, a Picker-Commonwealth Scholar Award, and a Merck Foundation Fellowship at Yaddo—all of which enabled us to pursue many of these and related ideas.

Nancy Van Devanter and Wafaa El-Sadr made it possible for us to interview participants in their research projects. At the HIV Center for Clinical and Behavioral Studies, Anke Ehrhardt provided unstinting support and opened the way for us to interview participants in the center's several studies.

A number of individuals offered critical assistance with preparation of the manuscript, including Lela Cooper, James Colgrove, Hannah Frisch, Ni-Tanya Nedd, Cydney Halpin, Michael Oks, and Shaira Daya. Others generously read the manuscript, including Renée C. Fox, Daniel Wolfe, Russell Hardin, Rebecca Stowe, D. Carleton Gajdusek, and Karl Wilder. Last, but by no means least, we wish to thank Charles Bieber and Jane Alexander.

MORTAL SECRETS

Secrets, Lies, and Private Life

"I tell the truth about half the time," he said. Tall, handsome, and intelligent, he worked in an AIDS service agency in New York. His candid acknowledgment about how he spoke to sexual partners was striking and surprising. He spoke as part of a study exploring how people adapt to the human immunodeficiency virus. Other men and women as well, in discussing the experience of being infected with HIV, repeatedly said that one of the hardest decisions they faced was whether to reveal the truth, to lie, or to speak in code to sexual partners and others in their lives.[1]

A series of questions arose. How do HIV-infected individuals make decisions about whom to tell? Why is disclosure, for many, among the most difficult aspects of being HIV positive? How do both HIV-infected and HIV-negative men and women view and approach the moral and practical dimensions of these dilemmas?

No one is an open book. We constantly face challenges of what to tell others about our lives. Do we announce when we are about to be divorced, have just been dumped by a lover, are seeing a therapist, or are depressed? When do we reveal that we have a potentially fatal disease? What does it mean to do so? We live in the post-therapeutic age, the age of confessional memoirs and television shows such as *Oprah* and *Jerry Springer,* in which strangers reveal secrets about formerly taboo matters such as incest—the more titillating, the better. Growing amounts of information about each of us are available every day through the Internet and computer databases. Contemporary society is in many ways increasingly open, with more topics fair game for discussion. Yet is everything in fact discussible? How does each of us chart the borders of our public and private selves in different settings? How do we map the boundaries of what is most secret, intimately ourselves, and what we reveal to others—whether near or far? In the anonymity afforded by contemporary urban society, and behind the hedges and fences of suburbia, secrets fill our lives.

Daily life is riddled with interactions that involve less than "the truth, the whole truth, and nothing but the truth." Communication is often veiled, oblique, and "slant," to use Emily Dickinson's term. For good or bad, secrets and lies are critical aspects of people's lives. Even in nature, among countless species of flora and fauna, deception and mimicry are essential to survival.

Secrets and lies permit human relationships to flourish, but can tear at their very core. The ability to hide information about ourselves can help us avoid unwanted intrusions from outsiders, but can also separate, isolate, and burden us. Lies can shield those we love from painful truths, but can also impede intimacy and friendship. How do we view secrets, deceptions, and lies, and how do our views contrast with our actions?

Revealingly, in recent years secrets and lies have emerged as important cultural themes. Films such as *Sex, Lies, and Videotape* and *Secrets and Lies* reflect the cultural anxiety and uncertainty about these realms. In the press, President Bill Clinton's affair with Monica Lewinsky raised further questions about what can and should be kept private, where the boundaries between the private and the public are and where they should be.

Sociologists have described how we, in the modern era, must manage information about ourselves. In his now classic *The Presentation of Self in Everyday Life,* Erving Goffman argued that in daily life all individuals operate as if on a theatrical stage, carefully presenting and framing information about themselves.[2] But we cannot always control knowledge about ourselves. Privacy may have grown in the nineteenth century with the rise of the bourgeoisie, but it is now under assault.

More recently, images of the closet—so central to contemporary gay sensibilities—have received attention in understanding individuals' experiences with secrecy and self-revelation. In *Epistemology of the Closet,* the postmodern critic Eve Kosofsky Sedgwick explored how "closetedness" has become a widely used metaphor in contemporary society. In daily life, individuals often "come out" about private aspects of themselves. "Coming out" involves an act—a "speech act," a performance that defines the self.[3]

The sexual revolution of the 1960s and 1970s radically transformed sexual practices and mores. Candor—letting it all hang out—became a virtue. Nevertheless, secrets continue to characterize even the most intimate sexual relationships. How much do we really know, or want to know, about our sexual partners? Can there be an ethics of sexual relationships, or is "sexual ethics" an oxymoron? Sex is, after all, a deeply rooted, hard-wired, prelinguistic realm of gratification.

We live in an ever more secular society in which the very nature and role of moral norms have become uncertain. Although Americans may attend religious services more frequently than the citizens of other economically advanced nations, the pervasive influence of religion has clearly declined. It is less possible now to speak of a moral consensus in everyday life. Instead, we acknowledge cultural diversities with their respective moralities, each of which claims our respect. Does this mean that anarchy prevails, or do the multiple moralities share some fundamental features? Do the roots of our moral promptings, though diverse, lead to some common points?

HIV provides a unique opportunity—a window to explore the territories of secrecy, morality, and silence. Encounters with HIV can tell us much about how we as individuals communicate about and view our bodies and most intimate selves—how we view and approach truth, lies, sex, and trust. The subject of sermons and commentaries, these issues are rarely studied systematically. Even less commonly do we hear the voices of those who confront these matters, gathered through careful interviews.

Sexual relationships—the physical intimacy of human interactions—involve a sharing of body parts and fluids, an opening of the self physically as well as psychologically. Such relationships often engender expectations of trust. Husbands and wives, boyfriends and girlfriends, lovers—all test, probe, and adjust these expectations over time. New relationships, dates, and courtships involve explicit or implicit expectations and negotiations. Inevitably, judgments must be made about whether a partner can be trusted and how much risk to take in the face of uncertainty. When assumptions about a partner's candor fail, individuals may feel profoundly disappointed, even betrayed. In the romantic ideal, trust deepens as relationships evolve— and vice versa. But, of course, that is not always the reality.

Even among sexual partners who share nothing but a desire for physical pleasure—one-night stands or encounters in bars, sex clubs, or baths—some rules of interaction surely apply. How do individuals permit themselves to feel free and aroused sexually, given the potential for harm? In the age of AIDS, these matters are crucial. For the uninfected, false steps or misjudgments could lead to the acquisition of a fatal disease. For the infected, deception could open the way to transmission of a lethal virus.

This exploration of disclosures about HIV also illuminates how individuals, discovering they are sick, integrate this knowledge into their lives and deepest notions of themselves to shape their identities. In Erving Goffman's powerful words, individuals must seek to "manage spoiled aspects" of their social and personal identities in a variety of contexts. They must conceal their condition, "pass" as untainted, or embrace the stigmatized characteristics.⁴ Finally, HIV furthers our understanding of the meanings of illness—how individuals enter a new role, that of being "sick."⁵

More than two decades have elapsed since the onset of the AIDS epidemic. Soon after physicians identified the first cases in 1981, it became clear that the agent responsible for the disease (even before that agent was isolated) could be transmitted through sexual intercourse and the sharing of needles by drug users. That AIDS was initially identified among gay men, drug users, and their sexual partners indelibly marked the environment in which the disease took shape in the United States. Fear of contagion merged with social hostility toward the infected. Gross acts of discrimination, occasionally accompanied by violence, punctuated the early years of the epidemic. At a time when both the health and the well-being of those infected and their sexual partners required openness and the possibility of self-disclosure, the social world fostered fear, secrecy, and a need to hide.

Now, more than twenty years after the first cases of HIV were reported, the disease continues to spread worldwide—at a rate of 16,000 new cases per day. Each year in the United States, 40,000 new cases arise. Efforts at prevention have stalled. Better ways of handling issues of disclosure, in conjunction with changed sexual practices, will be crucial to thwart the pandemic.

Such progress requires an appreciation of how those infected with HIV think about disclosing their infection and having sex. In our study, rather than speak *about* or even *for* those with HIV, we wanted to understand how those who are infected see their world and approach these issues. Our intent was to explore through narrative accounts how, in the extreme case of HIV and AIDS, people face questions of secrecy, morality, and trust.

Thus, we decided to interview men and women to explore how they confront these challenges. Specifically, we decided to map this landscape by conducting an ethnographic study—to obtain a "thick description," to use Clifford Geertz's term,⁶ of the world of disclosure among married couples, lovers, parents and children, friends and siblings, employees and employers, colleagues, and neighbors—addressing a broad set of critical questions. How do individuals decide whether, when, what, and to whom to disclose? Do they tell all partners or only some? And why? Do they disclose before, during, or after sex? What, if anything, do they feel they owe sexual partners? When they do not disclose, how do they behave sexually? What assumptions do they make about the role of truthfulness in sexual relationships? Do they make distinctions among those they view as anonymous sources of sexual gratification, those with whom they have ongoing relationships, and those they love? What rules and norms, if any, operate?

The answers to these questions have critical implications not only for

AIDS-prevention efforts but also for our understanding of deeper aspects of the human condition: what it is to live with stigma, secrecy, or deception. Moreover, what moral obligations do we have to intimates and strangers?

Theoretical Perspectives

Over the centuries, thinkers have wrestled with questions about truth, lies, deception, secrets, and trust. A range of views have emerged on the obligations of truth telling. These positions, though seemingly far from the world inhabited by people with HIV, represent intellectual scaffoldings for some of the issues that arise in the case of AIDS.

On the one extreme, as asserted by Immanuel Kant, lying can never be justified. "Truthfulness in statements is the formal duty of an individual to everyone, however great may be the disadvantage occurring to himself or to another."[7] The noted philosopher Sissela Bok, in her volume *Lying*—published just before the onset of the AIDS epidemic—rejected Kant's rigidity yet still set a very high bar for excusing lies (57–72). Those who were lied to had been "rendered powerless," their "very autonomy" subject to assault (18–19). She portrayed the consequences starkly. "Those who learn that they have been lied to in an important matter . . . are resentful, disappointed and suspicious. They feel wronged; they are wary of new overtures and they look back on their past beliefs and actions in the new light of discovered lies. They see that they were manipulated, that the deceit made them unable to make choices for themselves according to the most adequate information available, unable to act as they would have wanted to act had they known all along" (20).

For Bok, those who tell lies to shield others (i.e., for benevolent reasons) consider only the possibility of protecting those they seek to deceive and fail to recognize that the act of lying harms the broader fabric of social trust. Assaults on that fabric are cumulative and hard to reverse (24). Bok concluded by noting, "Trust and integrity are precious resources, easily squandered, hard to regain. They can thrive only on a foundation of respect for veracity" (249).

Given her antipathy to lying, it is striking that in her subsequent book, *Secrets,* turning to the ethics of concealment and revelation, she valued, above all, individuals protecting their privacy. "To be able to hold back some information about oneself," she noted, "or to channel it and thus influence how one is seen by others gives great power."[8] Just as lying represents a form of coercion, the inability to preserve secrecy makes one vulnerable to others. "To have no capacity for secrecy is to be out of control over how others see one; it leaves one open to coercion" (19).

But having argued for preserving secrecy, autonomy, and the protection of privacy, Bok also acknowledged that secrecy has its limits. Secrecy often conflicts with "the desire to share one's secret, to confide, to unburden, to reach out for greater intimacy" (37). Secrecy can also injure—linking it to some types of lying. "When the freedom of choice that secrecy gives one person limits or destroys that of others, it affects not only his own claims to respect, but theirs. Because it eludes interference, secrecy is central to the planning of every form of injury to human beings" (26).

In elucidating the moral implications of both lying and secrecy, Bok focused on how such behaviors enhance or subvert the possibility of men and women living together in communities of trust and respect for privacy. Only careful analysis can determine the extent to which concealment serves good or malevolent ends. Lying, on the other hand, can be tolerated only under the rarest of circumstances. For her, truth telling should guide our everyday behaviors.

Inevitably, the severity of Bok's strictures drew critics. David Nyberg, also a moral philosopher, challenged the moral centrality of truth telling and Bok's concerns about the personal and social harms caused by lying. In *The Varnished Truth,* he posed four questions: "What in the world is so awfully good about telling the truth all the time? Why should we feel obliged to excuse or justify every deception? Haven't we got the value of truth telling a little out of focus? Can it be that truth telling is really overrated?"[9]

Like Bok, Nyberg cherishes privacy and recognizes how important it is to the sense of dignity and decency. But unlike her, he argues that both privacy and communal life depend on something beyond truth telling. Indeed, balancing privacy and social civility satisfactorily "would be beyond reach without deception" (135). Deception can uniquely protect individuals from unwanted and unwarranted intrusions. Only deception softens the harsh edges of "the truth" and permits us to interact with those around us.

The force of his views becomes particularly clear in friendships. Like Bok, Nyberg sees trust as central to our relationships with friends—particularly intimate ones. "In friendship, what I entrust is myself . . . I rely upon you to look after me. Whatever happens in friendship then happens in an atmosphere of reciprocal trust" (141). But while Bok sees trust as requiring truth telling, for Nyberg, trust may in fact mandate that we deceive to protect those for whom we care. Trust entails the belief that those to whom we have made ourselves vulnerable will look after us. "That's a far greater and profounder gift than *mere* truth telling" (145). Nyberg reveals the depths of his separation from Bok by concluding his discussion with a quotation from Graham Greene's *Heart of the Matter.* "The truth, he thought, has never been of any real value to any human being—it is a symbol for mathematicians and philosophers to pursue. In human relationships kindness and lies are worth a thousand truths" (153).

Having set out to make the case that deception is integral to human well-being, Nyberg admits the limits of his own claims. Those forms of deception that place others at risk for injury fall outside the frame he painstakingly seeks to create. "I repudiate," he says, "all harmfully exploitative deceptions." Those forms of deception are "contemptible" (10).

The contemporary philosopher Thomas Nagel takes a similar stance. "The boundary between what we reveal and what we do not, and some control over the boundary," he writes, "are among the most important attributes of our humanity."[10] So important is the preservation of that boundary, says Nagel, that concealment is a condition of civilization. Ironically, he notes, we may feel compelled to lie when privacy is threatened, when the right to have secrets is challenged.

Over the past decade, social scientists and philosophers have further analyzed the role of trust in social and intimate settings. Why, in risky situations, do individuals trust each other? Some commentators have argued that individuals trust each other for instrumental reasons—anticipating direct gain in return. Others have emphasized the importance of noninstrumental bases for trust. Philosopher Russell Hardin argues for a notion of "trust as encapsulated interest." As he explains, "The trusted party has incentive to be trustworthy, incentive that is grounded in the value of maintaining the relationship into the further future. That is, I trust you because your interest encapsulates mine, which is to say, of course, that you have an interest in fulfilling my trust."[11] Thus, individuals trust after estimating the likelihood that others will reciprocate that trust or that others will meet their expectations of trust with regard to a particular behavior. Further along these lines, the psychologists Tom Tyler and Roderick Kramer have argued that individuals may trust a group to which they belong because they feel a sense of identity with its members, or a sense of moral or civic duty or commitment.[12]

The tone of the Bok-Nyberg debate, and the discussions of other philosophers, may seem a vast distance from the needs of those struggling to survive a lethal infection and social hostility. How do these divergent philosophical positions get played out amid the ambiguities of everyday life? Hence, we saw a need for ethnographies of how men and women wrestled with such issues. Such "thick descriptions," by definition, would have to focus with exquisite sensitivity on particular types and instances of truth telling, lies, secrecy, and trust—in order to illuminate most fully the range of nuances, variations, factors, and ramifications involved. Indeed, in our study, remarkably, we found that the words of individuals, many with less than a high school education, deepened and enriched our understanding of issues and complexities that have animated so much of past and contemporary moral discourse.

Protection of Self, Protection of Others, and the AIDS-Prevention Debate

The HIV epidemic has forced not only individuals but also policy makers and public health officials to confront matters of secrecy, trust, and truth. Even when explicitly abjuring the language of morality, their efforts to understand how people behave in the face of AIDS, as well as the public debate about how individuals should behave, have had to address these underlying psychological and moral quandaries.

From the epidemic's outset, controversies emerged over whether infected individuals had special duties to protect their uninfected sexual partners. In the early years, many concerned with HIV prevention rejected such claims. These opponents raised three objections, implicitly or explicitly. The first was pragmatic; the second, philosophical; the third, political.[13]

On a pragmatic level, opponents claimed that a public health policy that focused on the responsibility of people with HIV to behave in ways that protected the uninfected would in fact *increase* the risk of HIV transmission. Those who failed to protect themselves as a result of misguided expectations that they could trust their partners would be made more vulnerable. "Patients should be cautioned that safe sex strategies are always advisable despite arguments to the contrary from partners."[14]

This ethos of self-protection and "universal precautions" informed much of the AIDS-prevention effort in the first decade of the epidemic. Each man and woman had to be responsible for condom use. This obligation fell equally to the infected and the uninfected. As each person was responsible for his or her own health, no one was ultimately responsible for the health of the other. This implicit "code of the condom"[15] obviated any obligation to inform one's partner if one were infected. Thus, an educational pamphlet distributed by an AIDS service organization declared, "If you follow these safe sex guidelines, you don't need to worry about whether your partners know that you're positive. You've already protected them from infection and yourself from reinfection. Some guys need to get their HIV status out on the table. Just use your judgment about who you tell—there's still discrimination out there."[16]

Indeed, some felt the very concept of trust in intimate relationships was dangerous and had to be challenged. Based on an analysis of inner-city African-American women, Elisa J. Sobo concluded that "unsafe sex within a so-called faithful union helps a woman to maintain her state of denial about the risk of AIDS and her belief that her partnership is one of love, trust, and fidelity . . . AIDS risk denial is tied to monogamy ideals."[17] A harsh realism led Sobo to warn women about the dangers of trusting their male partners. It mattered little if these men were tricks, boyfriends, lovers, or husbands. Unprotected sex was always dangerous. Less tendentiously, some have asserted that a relationship could be a crucible of both security and risk.[18]

A second argument against trust and against claims that the infected had a duty to protect others was philosophical. This line of reasoning sought to displace the romantic notion of "love conquers all" with suspicion derived from the commercial exchange: caveat emptor—"let the buyer beware." Since HIV transmission largely occurred in consensual relationships that lacked expectations of truth telling, each individual bore the responsibility to protect himself or herself. Those who failed to protect themselves had no moral claim against those who infected them.[19] The possibility of the state intruding into the most intimate relationships fueled this philosophical perspective: if a moral duty to protect and disclose existed, it might lead to the imposition of criminal sanctions against unsafe sex.

A final objection to the claim that those with HIV infection had special responsibilities to prevent transmission was political. Threats to the privacy rights and the economic and social interests of the infected and those at risk of infection necessitated solidarity, and all efforts to distinguish between us and them, the tainted and the pure, those with HIV and those who had been spared, had to be rejected. Dangerously divisive attempts to impose special responsibilities on the infected would lead to a "viral apartheid." Divisions within the communities at risk would make it more difficult to develop broad-based social support for those affected by the epidemic. Social solidarity was best founded on the concepts of universal vulnerability to HIV and the universal importance of safer sex.

In the epidemic's first years, the ethic of self-protection rendered discussions of responsibility and self-disclosure all but impossible. The notion of self-protection had been accorded a central ideological role in the culture of AIDS-prevention efforts—especially among community-based organizations and local health departments most sensitive to the fears and concerns of those at highest risk for infection.

Nevertheless, some did argue that sexual partners were obligated to notify each other of their HIV status, drawing on the doctrine of informed consent.[20] Public health departments and the U.S. Centers for Disease Control and Prevention (CDC) devoted considerable attention to issues of partner notification in an attempt to assist those who were infected to warn their sexual partners about exposure to HIV. Nevertheless, in a 1995 review of AIDS-prevention efforts among drug users, Don Des Jarlais, a preeminent researcher in the field, noted, "Most programs that have urged intravenous drug users to use condoms thus far have focused on the self-protective efforts of condom use. Appealing to altruistic feelings of protecting others from HIV infection may be an untapped source of motivation for increasing condom use."[21]

Five years later, the Institute of Medicine, in its report, *No Time to Lose: The AIDS Crisis Is Not Over,* would conclude that public health efforts had overemphasized the prevention of HIV acquisition *by* uninfected individuals and had failed to recognize the critical importance of preventing HIV transmission *from* those who were infected. "Every new infection begins with someone who already is infected."[22] In the same year, a House of Representatives committee that had drafted a reauthorization bill for the Ryan White Care Act stated that "all counseling for HIV-infected individuals should emphasize that it is the duty of infected individuals to disclose their infected status to their sexual partners and others who they potentially may place at risk."[23] It was the obligation of agencies receiving funds under the act to provide counseling that emphasized that duty. Although many community-based organizations were already taking up that challenge, recognizing the limits of the earlier focus on self-protection, it was not clear how far this perspective had extended. The CDC itself was compelled to acknowledge the need for change. Its own review of state and city health departments' applications for AIDS-prevention funds in 1999 revealed that only one-third gave priority to efforts at working with HIV-positive individuals to reduce transmission. Thus, the federal health agency announced that it would expand prevention programs for those already infected "as a way to break the current rate of HIV transmission."[24]

Strikingly, the state of affairs has remained unsettled. In 2002 the *New York Times* reported AIDS educators' conclusion that a "new tactic" was necessary to prevent the spread of HIV: "educational campaigns encouraging people to take responsibility for not transmitting the virus."[25]

This evolving debate provided the context within which the men and women we interviewed for this study had to confront their own beliefs and understandings about concealment and disclosure.

Studies of Disclosure

Although not at the center of the vast social and behavioral research enter-prise that has surrounded the AIDS epidemic, the issue of self-disclosure of one's HIV infection has nonetheless drawn attention for more than a decade. Studies of disclosure conducted in the late 1980s and early to mid-1990s were primarily of gay men. In 1995 it was still possible for the authors of a thorough review of disclosure studies to lament the scant attention to women.[26]

In a trend that has continued, one of the first systematic studies of disclosure issues, involving only gay men, focused on the psychological burdens of secrecy and the potential benefits and costs of disclosure *for infected individuals*—but not on the moral issues affecting sexual partners. In setting the stage for their investigation, these San Francisco–based researchers noted, "Disclosure of one's HIV seropositivity to significant others is a double-edged sword. It may open up the opportunity to receive social support. However, it may also lead to added stress, due to stigmatization, discrimination, and disruption of personal relationships. Conversely, concealing one's HIV status from significant others may be stressful in itself and can interfere with obtaining and adhering to potentially critical medical treatments."[27]

The authors concluded that while disclosure could provide crucial sources of social support for infected gay men, important changes in the social climate would be necessary before it could be asserted that self-disclosure was "in the best interests of HIV-positive individuals."[28] Strikingly, the report contained not a word about how the issue of disclosure reflected questions of what sexual partners owed to each other concerning the potential risks of HIV transmission. Indeed, these early studies virtually ignored the meaning of silence to those who were infected and almost never discussed how those with HIV struggled with the moral, interpersonal, and practical implications of their silence.

We came to view the extant empirical studies of self-disclosure—both their focus and their methods—as profoundly limited and limiting. One of us (RK), a psychiatrist, had experience in medical anthropology and sociology and in ethnographic research methods. The other (RB), an ethicist, was concerned with public health policy and had experience in the conduct of oral histories. We believed that a fundamentally different approach was needed—that it was crucial to provide a research context within which men and women infected with HIV could describe how they understood the moral challenges posed by disclosure to sexual partners, family members, friends, and others in their lives. We were less concerned with counting responses—how many said what to whom, which dominated the literature—than with providing a broad yet detailed mapping of moral, social, and psychological decision making under conditions of extraordinary stress.

In short, we wanted to paint a picture of decisions about disclosure rather than prepare a numerical table. Only such an approach would allow us to convey the complex nuanced emotions of love, passion, raw lust, longing, hope, despair, and fear that powerfully shape decisions of whether to disclose to, deceive, or trust others about HIV. We have tried to present as fully as possible the voices of our informants and have chosen to allow these men and women to speak directly, intruding only by imposing structure and coherence to the multiplicity of perspectives elicited in our interviews.

Our approach has been informed by the work of Clifford Geertz and others in the social sciences that emphasizes the importance of understanding the perspectives of individuals within a given social or cultural context rather than imposing conceptual frameworks from without.[29] Carol Gilligan's work on the moral reasoning of boys and girls has demonstrated the power of probing moral choices from individuals' own perspectives and in their own words.[30] Even those who have been primarily concerned with ethics have begun to appreciate the relevance of how ethical issues emerge within specific contexts rather than in timeless, placeless arenas. In short, narrative has become increasingly important as a way of deepening our vision of the social and moral universe.[31]

In all, we interviewed 77 individuals (49 men, 28 women), 60 of whom (37 men, 23 women) were infected with HIV. Of the men, 30 were gay, 6 bisexual, and 13 heterosexual. Of the women, 26 were heterosexual—many of whom had no reason to suspect they might have been placed at risk by partners—and 2 were lesbian. Some of the men and women were living with or married to partners who were not infected. Of the infected men, 19 were gay, 13 heterosexual, 5 bisexual. Of the infected women, 22 were heterosexual and 1 was lesbian. In all, 41 of the interviewees were white, 26 African American, 8 Latino, and 2 Asian/Pacific Islander. All but one lived in New York.

We recruited participants in several ways: through a study of gay men with HIV, being conducted at our institution; a study of heterosexual couples of mixed HIV status; an infectious disease clinic at a large inner-city hospital that treated men and women of color, most of whom were injecting-drug users or their sexual partners; and advertisements in gay magazines.

To identify and describe the range of views and meanings of disclosure among individuals who confront HIV, we selected this sample to be representative of the major groups affected and infected by HIV: male and female injecting-drug users and their sexual partners—whether heterosexual, lesbian, or gay—and gay men.

This comparatively large number of voices could create a blizzard-like experience for the reader. Although we could have simplified our presentation and excluded some participants, all those we interviewed had something to add to an understanding of issues of disclosure. Their words add a degree of richness that would have been lost had we restricted our account. Still, some individuals appear more frequently here than others and hence serve to anchor our examination. In presenting the words of these men and women, we have changed names and some identifying details to protect their privacy.

We were aware of how difficult it might be for individuals with HIV to disclose to us behaviors that placed others at risk. We made every effort to create a context of candor. Some readers may wonder, however, whether individuals would divulge to us what they had hidden from others. We took a number of steps to enhance the prospects for open discussion. Our Institutional Review Board–approved study was confidential and could be anonymous. Individuals could provide us with only a first name or a pseudonym if they preferred. A federal Certificate of Confidentiality protected our work from compelled disclosure in legal proceedings. Yet whatever the pledge of confidentiality in research, resistance to admitting to socially undesirable behavior could make candor difficult. It is thus all the more remarkable that among those we interviewed, some acknowledged that they had engaged in behavior that placed their sexual partners, even spouses or long-term lovers, at risk. How they understood, explained, justified, or rationalized their choices provides insights about a more pervasive phenomenon—exposure to HIV by partners who deceive. Nevertheless, it is possible that we recruited individuals who in fact were more inclined than others to reveal their HIV status to sexual partners or who portrayed themselves as being more open. Thus, the frequency of nondisclosure in this sample might represent a floor, or lower bound, of such behavior.

Our interviews ranged from one to two hours and were tape recorded and transcribed verbatim. Each interview transcript was read and analyzed by both of us to maintain consistency. (See the appendix for the interview guide.) Data were content-analyzed, informed by grounded theory,[32] that is, by techniques of "constant comparison," in which data from different contexts are compared for similarities and differences, in order to understand the factors that shaped participants' experiences. As we read the interviews we sought to identify core categories (e.g., instances of disclosure or nondisclosure to lovers, children, siblings, and other family members). We then examined principal subcategories and the ranges and variations within these categories.

We conducted the interviews in the mid-1990s, fourteen years after the AIDS epidemic had begun and a full decade after HIV testing became possible. Some of those we interviewed had known for years that they were infected. Others had only recently been tested. Since the epidemic's first years, much had changed. The Americans with Disabilities Act provided some formal legal protection for those with AIDS and asymptomatic HIV infection. The politics of HIV had shifted in a myriad of ways from the presidencies of Ronald Reagan and George H. W. Bush to that of Bill Clinton. Nevertheless, the legacy of the epidemic's first decade, characterized by shameful neglect, had profoundly marked the lives and consciousness of those whom we interviewed—fueling fears of stigmatization.

By the mid-1990s the clinical prospect for those with HIV had altered as well. The management of the opportunistic infections due to HIV had progressed markedly but slowly since the 1980s. Therapeutic interventions had controlled some of the diseases associated with AIDS—most notably *Pneumocystis carinii* pneumonia (PCP), which was often fatal, and cytomegalovirus retinitis, a cause of blindness. What had not changed was the prognosis for most people with HIV infection. Hopes that AZT (azidothymidine; zidovudine)—licensed in 1987 as the first antiretroviral drug—could slow the course of disease or delay the progression from HIV to AIDS had proved illusory.[33] By the mid-1990s it could still be said that AIDS equaled death.

In 1996, therapeutic advances altered the clinical prospects for those with HIV and AIDS.[34] The discovery of the protease inhibitors and the advent of potent combination therapies using an array of antiretrovirals (known as HAART, highly active antiretroviral therapy) radically altered the immediate and short-term prognoses for those with HIV. Many men and women close to dying were given new hope.[35] Those with less advanced disease were given a reprieve. Yet uncertainty still hovered. No one could know for sure how long the new therapies would elude the threat of HIV. Nor did the medications work for everyone. Still, for those living with infection in the late 1990s and the first years of the new millennium, the link between HIV and mortality had been attenuated.

Despite such changes, the words we heard from men and women struggling with their mortal secrets remain critically relevant, for several important reasons. Although AIDS is now perceived as a chronic disease, it is still believed to be ultimately fatal. It can be treated but not cured. Moreover, although the suppression of viral loads (the amount of virus in the blood) achieved by new therapies dramatically decreases the risks of transmission,

HIV can still be passed between sexual partners and those who share injection equipment.

The new therapeutic era has not changed the significance or difficulty of self-revelation. Indeed, research with which we have been involved makes clear that HIV disclosure remains an enormous, central, and defining problem.[36] The friends and family members to whom individuals disclose still cry and experience great emotional distress. Some family members fear that young children will become infected through close contact. As a result, many, especially women, remain highly closeted about their infection, telling no one or only one or two people in their lives. The secret of HIV is kept from children, family members, and even health care providers. Many do not tell all of their sexual partners.

Frequently, those in treatment try to hide their medications, particularly at work. To take pills in front of others—even those who know of one's HIV infection—can be difficult. Nevertheless, HAART can force unwitting divulgence. Disclosure often now occurs through the apparent side effects of the medications rather than visible symptoms of the disease itself. In the epidemic's first years, some individuals "looked sick" because of the wasting syndrome or Kaposi sarcoma—lesions that occurred as a part of HIV. Now physical symptoms such as lipodystrophy—the maldistribution of body fat leading to hump back and hollowed cheeks—tell the story. As a consequence, some infected men and women have stayed in jobs they would otherwise leave, simply because they feel that their current environment is "safe" whereas future employers and work settings might not be.

Efforts to hide one's infection and the use of antiretroviral medications may have a significant impact on adherence to these exacting medical regimens. To preserve their secrecy, individuals may feel compelled to skip doses. But such self-protective efforts may lead to the development of viral resistance to therapy, an outcome with critical implications for the effectiveness of treatment—and for public health, since drug-resistant strains of HIV can be transmitted to sexual and needle-sharing partners.

Improved treatments for HIV pose additional dangers, as recent studies have suggested that the reduced threat of HIV may lead young gay men to reduce their vigilance. An increase in sexually transmitted diseases (STDs) makes it clear that such men are having unprotected sex.[37] A study in Baltimore, Chicago, Los Angeles, and Pittsburgh concluded, "Lessened concern about HIV transmission due to [HAART] was strongly associated with sexual risk taking." Weariness of the demands of safer sexual practices, "safer sex fatigue," among infected and uninfected men increases risky behaviors. Furthermore, such changes in risk taking are occurring at the very moment that those with HIV infection experience increased vitality during their now extended lives.[38] Among men in New York City, for example, one survey found that 46 percent of all respondents had had unprotected anal sex during the prior six months; 30 percent had had such sex with a pick-up or one-night stand; 25 percent had had such sex for money, food, or shelter.[39] In San Francisco between 1994 and 1997, rates of unprotected anal sex increased most markedly among those less than 25 years of age.[40] A 2001 review in the *American Journal of Public Health* drew the only possible conclusion: "The HIV epidemic among [men who have sex with men] is continuing at a very high level." This was especially so for African Americans, those who used both injectable and noninjectable drugs, and those who were less educated. In a stark comparison, the analysis concluded that HIV prevalence rates among urban men who engaged in homosexual behavior are "similar to those for sub-Saharan Africa."[41] The rates of new infection among poor African-American women are even more disturbing. Among adolescents, African-American females have some of the highest HIV infection rates in the United States.[42] The seriousness of the situation is compounded by the extent to which drug-resistant strains of HIV are being transmitted in the newly infected.[43]

Confronting this ongoing pattern of HIV transmission requires a renewed consideration of the importance of disclosure. But disclosure requires that individuals know they are infected. For years, public health officials have assumed that in the United States more than one-third of the 900,000 who have HIV are unaware of their condition. Among young urban men who have sex with men, a majority who are infected do not know that they harbor the virus. More alarming, in a report issued by the CDC in 2001, only 7 percent of infected African-American young men knew they had HIV. In the CDC study, 55 percent stated that they had not been tested because they were "scared to learn the results."[44] Fear still shapes the epidemic.

The accounts presented in this volume, although they emerged from a particular moment in the history of the AIDS epidemic, shed light on the most enduring matters in human relationships—love, truth, morality, desire, and trust. The voices of these men and women elucidate how human beings face each other in the shadow of illness and death. These tales also document an important moment in cultural, social, and medical history, a time of shifting sexual and personal mores and of intense political challenge to the very notion of mutual obligation. Here, we can glimpse people's innermost lives as they struggle with the most fundamental issues of our time.

GETTING TESTED

Uncovering the Truth

Deciding to get tested for HIV can profoundly change one's life. The decision may involve a protracted process of weighing the risks and benefits of learning the truth in the light of possible discrimination, and the burdens of being diagnosed with a fatal disease. For the individuals in our study, how they decided whether to be tested and how they reacted to their diagnoses shaped how they then faced questions of whether to tell partners, families, and friends. Their choices reflected their appraisals of the extent of their own risk, their capacity to confront how their own behaviors had exposed them to HIV, and the degree to which they needed or were able to hide from the truth by self-deception.

Views of the HIV antibody test have changed over time. The test itself did not become available until 1985, four years after the first reports of AIDS by the U.S. Centers for Disease Control and Prevention. Initially used in blood banks to detect the presence of HIV and to prevent transfusion-associated AIDS, the antibody test quickly spread as a diagnostic tool to inform those who were not symptomatic whether they harbored a lethal and transmissible virus.

Most public health officials viewed the HIV test as permitting the infected to know that they could, even if inadvertently, transmit infection to others.[1] In 1985 the CDC recommended that all individuals who had either engaged in risky behaviors or received blood transfusions undergo voluntary testing.[2] To make such testing less threatening, the CDC called for the strictest measures of confidentiality and for protection of the infected from discrimination. The CDC also gave funds to local health departments to establish anonymous testing centers that would free those seeking testing from the need to provide any identification.

Yet the test alarmed gay leaders and the first generation of AIDS activists.[3] The lack of available therapy for those who tested positive and a prevailing hostile social climate provided ready reasons to avoid testing. Since universal precautions urged both the infected and uninfected to adopt sexual practices that could preclude viral transmission, many argued that no public health reason existed to seek testing.

Early in the epidemic in New York City, where our interviews took place, the Department of Health adopted a public posture that reflected the gay community's concerns, and in so doing set itself apart from many of the nation's public health officials.[4] In fact, the department's AIDS hot line discouraged callers from seeking HIV antibody testing. It was in the face of such attitudes that individuals who believed themselves at risk had to confront the question of whether, in the absence of frank disease, they should find out whether they had this lethal infection.

Then, in the late 1980s, the social climate surrounding testing began to change. Early diagnosis now appeared to offer a clinical benefit for infected individuals, through prophylactic treatment against opportunistic infection.[5] The public health claim that testing could serve as an adjunct to counseling in assisting individuals to alter their behaviors became a convention, even in New York. Finally, the mandate that all gay couples use condoms all the time regardless of HIV status began to seem too burdensome.

Finding Out

Individuals varied widely in why they got tested. Some had their blood assayed as a precautionary measure to make sure they were healthy, others to avoid the necessity of condom use or because they wanted to have a child. People also sought testing to discover whether they had acquired the infection from a partner. Still others did not choose to be screened but had knowledge of their HIV infection thrust upon them. No matter how the journey began, those who learned they were infected had to confront profoundly transforming knowledge about themselves.

Almost always, apprehension surrounded the process of getting tested—fears of being found out by others and of learning of dangers in one's body. Nevertheless, many sought testing anyway since they could not tolerate the uncertainty of not knowing. Gary, a white gay man in his early forties who said he used to be "Mr. Safe Sex," had assumed he was at low risk because he was the insertive rather than the receptive partner in anal intercourse with his lover of sixteen years. Even so, he decided to get tested soon after that became possible.

> Very early in the epidemic, I was tested, and we were kind of afraid to go any place in Manhattan, so we schlepped out to Jamaica, Queens, to be tested.

> And this clinic had just opened, and I remember there was nothing in this office except one poster, which said, "One dumb move." I was not expecting to be positive at all because for the most part I'm a top, and it seemed like bottoms were getting this disease.

Sadly, he was wrong.

Recognition that a history of high-risk sex or drug use could cause infection also fueled the anxiety about undergoing the blood assay. Emanuel, a 37-year-old white heterosexual, had abandoned drug use and would eventually get a master's degree in social work. He chose to be tested two years after entering a drug-treatment program.

> After having run the streets of New York City and nearly lost my life several times, just hustling for drugs and doing that whole street scene all them years, I thought I escaped this bullet. A couple of years later I got tested. I got into therapy to try to prepare myself. I was real anxious about taking the test.

Emanuel had gone to get tested, afraid that his worst fears would be confirmed, but others denied or downplayed, even sought to ignore, the very symptoms that might suggest they were infected. Ramon, a married African-American injecting-drug user, said, "I started to get some night sweats. I didn't really think it was anything serious. So I just decided to get tested, let me just go and clear my mind and make sure that I'm okay. And I wasn't." In fact, he later had the test repeated to make sure it was correct.

For others, the possibility of infection could seem very remote. For example, Sherri, a 31-year-old white heterosexual physician, decided to test herself as a prelude to undergoing hepatitis treatment that would affect her immune system.

> During my internship, I had a very bad needle stick and got hepatitis C. For a long time I had been thinking about testing myself for HIV. I actually raised the issue with my gastroenterologist, and he just didn't think it was a good idea. But when treatment first came out for hepatitis C—alpha-interferon—I thought, since it's an immune modulator, I ought to know my HIV status. So I tested myself, never thinking that it was going to come out positive. At the time I was living in a five-flight walk-up, and this thing came back in my mailbox, and I thought I was going to die. It literally took my breath away. But I made it up the stairs and called my therapist.

Some tested to see whether they could abandon the strictures of "safer sex," which mandated that condoms be used in every sexual encounter. Yet they, too, could be surprised by unwanted news. Sergio, a 37-year-old gay

Latino who worked for an international communications corporation, said,

> I went with my partner. The two of us had been together for a few years then, and up to that point had been practicing safe sex. But we decided now we'd get tested and if we're both negative then we can sort of let the spirits run wild. And we got tested. I kind of suspected I might be positive because I had a fairly interesting history in celebrating my sexuality.

Regardless of the self-perception of being at low risk for infection, an individual could choose to undergo testing as a result of news that a current or former lover was infected. These self-perceptions need not have entailed self-deception. Ernest, a white heterosexual screenwriter, was 38 years old when a former girlfriend with whom he had had sex only once alerted him to his risk.

> I received a letter from an old girlfriend of mine that she now had AIDS, so I went and got a test. I'd probably once or twice mentioned testing to my doctor when I'd go in for a check-up . . . He would say, "No, no, unless you've had any high-risk behavior." And I really hadn't. I'm not an IV drug user. I had to wait over the weekend. But I went and got a test the following week and it came out positive.

An impending marriage or plans to have children could also set the stage for testing. Jane, a young married Jewish woman, believed she had nothing to fear. But her husband, who wanted to have children, was anxious. Repeatedly in the late 1980s, the popular media headlined the universality of risk: "Now no one is safe," the stories proclaimed.

> I tested because my husband and I had decided to start a family. When he had tested negative I pretty much assumed I must be negative as well. When he suggested it, I'd actually gotten angry at him that he even dared to suggest I might have been exposed to it. But I discussed it with one of my friends who told me she had been tested, so I thought maybe it's not such a bad idea just for our peace of mind. My doctor didn't want to do it. He said, "Just go and get tested at one of the anonymous sites." At the anonymous sites you had to make appointments, and it's just a hassle, so finally I insisted that my doctor do it, and he asked me a few questions, and said, "You're really not at risk, I'll call you if the results are negative, and I'll ask you to come in if they were positive," which was a stupid thing to do, actually. And I said, "Fine." We had to bring the blood over to the Department of Health, and about nine days later or so I got a phone call at the office from the doctor's nurse. She asked me to come in, that the doctor wanted to see me right away. So, I knew.

In trying to understand how she might have been infected, Jane thought of a man with whom she had slept ten times before her marriage, who had a history of drug use.

For individuals who did not choose to be tested but had to undergo screening as blood donors or applicants for insurance, learning of the diagnosis and that they had been at risk literally came out of nowhere—a bitter surprise. Since 1983 the CDC had strongly urged those who had engaged in behaviors that might have increased their risk of AIDS not to donate blood. Screening for HIV, from mid-1985, was designed either to identify those who, despite such warnings, attempted to donate or to detect HIV in those who had no reason to believe they were at risk. Jim, a 36-year-old white computer programmer who had had several homosexual encounters in the past but was now married, demonstrated how minimizing the significance of past behavior could inform the process of self-deception. "I got a test because I was donating blood to a relative of my wife who was going in for an operation. And since I have type O blood it was thought that I could donate safely to her."

Life insurance companies required testing as part of the underwriting process, to exclude those who would pose an additional burden on the insured risk pool. Many who had reason to think they were infected avoided the embarrassment of rejection and being "found out" by forgoing coverage. Others, who thought themselves at no risk or denied their risk, were startled to learn otherwise. A young married physician, for example, was "stunned" —despite having had sex with men—when his application for life insurance was turned down and he was told, upon inquiry, that he was infected with HIV.

Starting in 1985, the U.S. military began to screen in order to exclude those with HIV infection from the service. Despite his bisexuality, Patrick, a white police officer—who was a 32-year-old reserve officer when he was tested—was utterly unprepared for his HIV infection. Denial shielded him from acknowledging his risk.

> I was going from one branch of the reserves, the Marine Corps, and was transferring to a Green Beret unit upstate. I don't know if I signed a statement to get tested. Even if I did, I still would have thought I'm okay—even though I knew I had risky behavior. I would just deny it because I was too healthy at that point. I knew my past: a lot of street prostitutes, male and female. Maybe twice I tried IV drugs. I got sick as a dog from them, and thank God I never went back to them. Sexually, I'd been on the circuit—frisky, risky. I present a very heterosexual appearance. At that point it kind of caught me—a blind-side

punch. They sent me a letter saying to come down to Fort Hamilton. That's where they told me.

Prisoners, too, had little choice about testing. "I got locked up in '88," said Donald, an uninfected bisexual African American in his early forties who later lived in a shelter. "They don't even have to ask you, because you're locked up. You automatically got to take that test."

Finally, some women learned they were infected because their children were diagnosed with HIV or full-blown AIDS. Thus, simultaneously, these women had to confront the facts that their children were critically ill and that they themselves harbored a lethal virus. Regina, a 41-year-old hetero-sexual African American with a history of drug use, discovered her HIV in-fection and that of her 22-month-old son as part of his diagnostic workup. She experienced a double blow, accompanied by palpable guilt.

> He started getting sick and they found out that he was HIV, and so they found out that I was, too. I was devastated. The thought that my lifestyle was caus-ing him not to have a life was really hard. It would have been much easier for me had his life not been involved. It was really very rough. I tried to take my own life. I didn't want to have to go through the things that they were saying. I definitely didn't want to see my child go through this.

Reactions: A World Turned Upside Down

Clearly, individuals differed in how they initially reacted, from denial to shock or even attempted suicide. The diagnoses could represent the threat of a series of losses—of health, social standing, identity, and life itself.

A very few heard the diagnosis with little apparent reaction. They knew what they had done and how widespread the epidemic was, and they re-ported that, even if disappointed, they weren't surprised. Larry, a 49-year-old white gay man who was an emigré from New Zealand, had recently started a relationship when he found out.

> I was fully expecting to be positive because of my sexual activity. I wasn't con-scious of having a bad reaction. I was already depressed from grieving for my friend. So I really can't say that I was aware of having a reaction to the news of being HIV positive. Subconsciously, there was a bit of disappointment. Maybe I hoped I got away with it.

Others believed a positive result had to be a mistake. Jim, who had had ho-mosexual relationships in the past but was now married, said, "I was con-vinced that there was simply an error. I'd have to say there was a little bit of fear, but I was very much in control of myself, simply because I was sure that there was an error."

Most, however, were utterly overwhelmed when learning they were infected, though intellectually not surprised. George, a 37-year-old white gay man diagnosed when he was 30, had moved to New York from San Francisco to begin his doctoral studies in clinical psychology just days after learning about his HIV status. He responded to his diagnosis by desperately seeking to reassert control, trying to master what was known about AIDS. "Everybody has their own kind of defense as a way of dealing with it. Mine was trying to focus on information."

A diagnosis of HIV often profoundly disrupted individuals' views of themselves and their place in the world. Camille, an Asian/Pacific Islander in her mid-thirties who was infected by a heterosexual partner, had no reason to believe she was at risk.

> A counselor took me in the room, and said, "I'm sorry to tell you, your test came back positive." I just remember staring at her. I just felt like my world just dropped to the floor. I was stunned, in disbelief. Minutes were going by. I was in shock. She was talking to me, but I couldn't hear. I can only retain basically one thing out of the whole counseling period. The only thing I heard was, "Do what it is you want to do with your life from this day on." To me, that was like a death sentence. I was on the other side. When I didn't think that I carried the virus, I was just like everybody else. Those stories in the newspaper are a curiosity. You bypass it. It doesn't make any real impact on us until we're actually affected by it.

Jane, the woman who got tested because she wanted to have children, also felt a radical disjunction in her life. "I remember I went home, and everyone on the subway looked bizarre, and it just seemed like everything had ended. My whole life as I knew it was over, and everything that was still functioning seemed strange to me." Ellen, a 27-year-old white heterosexual journalist who presumed she had been infected through a blood transfusion, said, "It just seemed like a bad TV movie."

Some experienced acute numbness and helplessness. Gladys, a 45-year-old heterosexual African American who was a business manager at a telephone company, sought testing when the man she had lived with for years—a former drug user—finally acknowledged during a hospitalization that he had AIDS. She said, "I stayed numb for a long time. There were no tears. Even the bitterness wasn't there. I just didn't know what to do."

Diagnosis could shatter a sense of the coherency not only of the world but of identity as well. When military officials told Patrick, the marine reservist, that he was infected, they disrupted both his life and the elaborate pattern of secrets and deceptions he had created.

> I just was crying and busted out of the door and started running, I just wanted to run, and that's how I coped with AIDS. I'm going out the gate: "What the fuck am I going to do?" My image of myself was totally shattered. "How am I going to fucking tell anybody? How am I going to live with this? What if people find out?"

The virus could alter one's sense of the body itself. Gary, the gay man who was surprised at his infection because he had always been the insertive partner during unprotected anal sex, said, "I have this viral infection that isn't going to go away. It's part of me, part of my body. That freaks me out." The body itself could feel sullied. "I feel," said one gay man, "like damaged goods." Van, an infected 34-year-old white gay man—in a relationship with Paul, who was uninfected—added, "I just felt real sleazy about myself at that point—dirty."

For those who had struggled to overcome addictions to drugs, an HIV diagnosis could feel like a betrayal of all their efforts. Keith, a 41-year-old heterosexual African American who worked for a phone company, reported,

> At the time I had a little over six years in recovery, and had put my life together and done all the things that've been asked of me, because I used to be a rebel. I was a month away from getting remarried at the time, I got a whole future ahead of me, and we were talking about having kids. And bang.

The diagnosis could also be seen as the loss of a future. Ginger, a 37-year-old white woman living with her boyfriend, learned she was infected when she was 29, a few years after becoming sober from injecting-drug use. With her diagnosis, she felt life's options had been taken away.

> Part of me feels I'm missing, I'm not able to dream that dream when two people fall in love. What's the dream? Maybe we'll get married, have kids. Maybe we'll retire together and spend a wonderful life together. And I just got to go, "Well, maybe we'll have a couple of nice years together. Maybe we'll enjoy today."

And, of course, HIV diagnosis forced many individuals to confront their mortality. Tony, a 36-year-old white bisexual, had in the past injected cocaine, then returned to college to study anthropology. After his diagnosis, he felt for the first time a limitation on his life. "I knew that I was at high risk, but to me it was one of those things that happens to other people. It wouldn't happen to me: I'm immortal. That was a big blow." Indeed, many felt the diagnosis meant that death was imminent. These reactions, though particularly acute before the advent of powerful combination therapies in the mid-1990s, persisted even later. Andrew, a 55-year-old gay chef, said, "In my mind I started to think, how many days do I have left?" Similarly, Emanuel, the former drug user who became a social worker, noted, "I started feeling like my life is over, like it wasn't no use going on. Doomed to die. I couldn't see myself living past a month. It was like, 'Well, I'm going to die tomorrow.'" Darryl, a 36-year-old heterosexual African American, was a former drug user and had spent many years in jail as a result of drug-related charges. He thought of the loss his death would represent to his son.

> When I left the office, I was just thinking about my son. I just thought about not being able to see him grow up. I was in my car just riding, feeling lost, similar to the feeling that I had when I was using drugs. I was just by myself, wandering in the streets, lost, a lot of thoughts coming into my mind, rushing through my mind, and I just drove. I just drove.

In extreme cases, as we have seen, thoughts of suicide arose. Ali, a 51-year-old heterosexual African American, had used heroin and cocaine for years. He was 46 when he learned his diagnosis. Still using drugs at the time, he said, "It was something that I couldn't accept. I even contemplated suicide. I tried to drive my car into a tree once, and for some reason God wasn't ready to take me out, so I missed the tree."

Deciding Whether to Disclose

As they began to confront the enormity of what they had learned about themselves, infected men and women immediately had to face a second set of issues with profound implications: whom to tell. Craig, a 27-year-old white gay man, was a hairdresser and former male prostitute who had learned he was infected when he was 17. He remarked, "Knowing that you have it and living with it is the most difficult. I think the list goes on, and number two would be disclosure: who to let know, when to let them know, how to let them know, and what their reaction is going to be."

Like Craig, those who were newly diagnosed had to contemplate how best to avoid the pain of social rejection. In so doing, they had to balance the desire for support against the concern that disclosure could prompt the very rejection, isolation, and discrimination that they feared. William, now in his mid-forties—a white "gay man who got married"—was engaged when he learned of his HIV infection, having hidden his homosexual past from his fiancée. His counselor warned him against impulsively reaching out to others, saying, "You must think very carefully about this before you discuss it with anyone. Many people feel the need to tell somebody right away, they need somebody to talk to. That's fine, find somebody to talk to, but find a professional person. Do not tell your family, your friends. Sit with it." "It was," William said, "very good advice." Sergio, the gay man working for an international communications corporation, simply urged caution. "If I were advising someone, I would say, think very hard about what reward you might get, recognizing that the consequences could be really horrible."

Among the most difficult aspects of HIV disclosure was that it ordinarily required telling the story of how one got infected—divulging homosexuality, use of drugs, or sexual encounters with individuals who might be perceived as having shady pasts. When Sherri, the physician, told the physicians treating her about her HIV infection, she felt she was revealing more than a clinical fact. "It was hard for me, and it was hard for them, just to tell my story again, just another rehashing of everything," particularly that she had had an affair with a "gambler" who she thought infected her.

Consequently, individuals had to decide *how* to tell—how to frame the information and construct a narrative about their infection. Many tried to cast the information as positively as possible. Howard, for example, a 51-year-old white teacher living in Philadelphia, was direct, viewing disclosure as the norm among gay men. "I was always real careful when I'd tell people, that when I said it, I was coming from a positive place. I didn't want them to hear something negative." Camille believed she could ease the response of those with whom she was sexually involved by telling them about how it was possible to be intimate without incurring the risk of transmission. "The more information I provide on my side, the more it helps that other person deal with the information differently."

Like Camille, others sought to "educate," in part to avoid responsibility for the behaviors sexual partners might be willing to engage in. Ginger, for example, the former injecting-drug user who felt HIV had deprived her of her dreams for the future, had a standard spiel.

> I have this magical way, when I tell someone, anyone, even a date, family member, friend, whatever, I immediately want to jump right into almost being a clinician, saying, "Okay, now, blah blah blah, these are the facts, these are the figures, blah blah blah. This is an issue that you need to spend some time thinking about. I in no way want to influence your thoughts on this, so I encourage you, if you're even interested, to get as much information as you can from all the sources that you can, not just from me."

She wanted her partners to learn on their own the parameters of safer sex—
with its inherent uncertainties.

> I really don't like to proceed with, "Oh, by the way, this is what safe sex is,"
> because I prefer that the guy find out from a different source, I really do. I'm
> just more comfortable with that. If anything happens in the future I don't
> want him to turn around and say, you know, "She said if I use a condom with
> a hole in it it's safer sex."

Like the decision about what to tell, the decision about *whom* to tell was
neither simple nor straightforward. Some saw decisions about disclosure as
involving a deliberative process; others, as requiring an almost instinctive
sense of what felt right. For example, Claudio, a 44-year-old Latino drug
counselor who had been infected through prior drug use, said, "I trusted in
my feeling. I went with my gut feeling, taking the risk."

The willingness to reveal one's infection could change over time, the revelation becoming less difficult with each successive disclosure. Sam, an infected 37-year-old white gay man who worked as a respiratory therapist, explained, "I think certain people have no business knowing, like your
employer, for example, and people that could use that information against
you. With more experience, it becomes easier. Now, pretty much I have no
qualms about telling people." The patterns of disclosure were so obviously
varied, and reflected so many different needs, that even those who were negative could appreciate the complexities involved. As one uninfected woman
said, "It's one of those things where everybody's got to do what works for
them. For some people disclosing is very helpful and for some people it's
not."

Decisions about disclosure often reflected more general personal characteristics. Jim, for example, said, "I'm not a private person. I tend to tell
people. So I told the people I work with." Similarly, Roberta, a 46-year-old
heterosexual African American who was infected, saw herself as generally
outspoken. "I just feel more open about myself now than I did before. I never
did bite my tongue." Some revealed their HIV infection because they saw it
as an essential part of their identity—something that had to be disclosed to
the people in their lives. As Howard, the gay teacher, said,

> Being positive is very much part of who I am. And if I'm going to have sex with
> somebody, they need to know some things about me and who I am. And that
> is one of the very important ones. Why is it important that they know I'm from
> New York? I live in Philadelphia. I love telling people I'm from New York. I love
> telling people I have HIV. I love telling people I'm a teacher. It's just a part of

my whole makeup. And I think if you're going to have sexual relations with somebody, I want to know where they're from. I want to know things about them. Just knowing the person you're with.

Conversely, others said they hesitated to tell because they were by nature "private" and kept things to themselves. Maria, a 31-year-old heterosexual Latina who worked as a secretary, spoke about the four years that had passed since she learned she was infected.

I'm definitely independent in that I'm more of a private person. I don't like to burden other people. I think, especially now when it has not really affected my life physically, that if I don't think about it that much, then life is normal. Right now it's kind of like maintenance, and if I had diabetes or something, you just keep the medication up, keep going because fortunately, like I said, I don't have anything.

It is noteworthy that she—and others as well—suggested a kind of magical thinking: if they did not think about being infected, if they did not disclose their situation, or if they minimized the significance of their diagnosis, they could prevent themselves from becoming sicker.

Finally, as we shall see in the next chapter, decisions about disclosure could be profoundly affected by economic and emotional dependency. Many women, especially poor women, feared that disclosure to male partners could result in loss of financial support, making the cost of candor very high, "countering the more usual tendencies of women to reveal intimate information."[6]

For a few, fears and shame led to a decision to tell few, if any, people. For example, Wilma, a 38-year-old heterosexual African American who was homeless, had learned of her infection when giving birth to her son and had delayed disclosing, telling no one for five years. In the end she told only one person. "Nobody knows I'm HIV positive except one person now: my sister." Similarly, Dolores, a 43-year-old heterosexual African American, "the black sheep" in her family, told no one until she could no longer hide it. Only the man who infected her knew.

I didn't tell anybody for over two and a half years. I didn't tell my kids, my mother, nobody. For two and a half years, I just lived with it, and this was between me and him. But then when he started getting sick, my kids were coming round. They'd say, "Look . . ." And I'd say, "No." Then he died from AIDS, and I said, "I'm HIV positive." But for two and a half years I lived with it just between us. I didn't tell nobody.

Some took their secret to the grave. Steve, an uninfected 33-year-old white gay man, owner of a pet store, lived with his HIV-positive partner and described himself as highly conscientious, "a goody two shoes." He said with dismay, "There's people who tell everybody, and there's people who tell nobody. I know somebody who didn't tell anyone, and he died and that was it. He went away and everybody said, 'Where did he go?'"

SEXUAL PARTNERS

Sex, Love, and Disclosure

To be infected with HIV is to face a moral and psychological challenge: how honest to be with sexual partners. The infected men and women with whom we spoke had to decide whether and whom to inform—only current partners or those from the past as well? Some felt morally obligated to tell the truth all the time. Others felt no obligation to tell anyone and were concerned only for their own well-being and sexual gratification. But between these two opposing moral worlds, men and women generally struggled to find a course that both protected themselves in a potentially punitive world and avoided injuring others. In striving to find their way, they exposed some central dilemmas of moral decision making in the most intimate of contexts.

Sexual relationships take on radically diverse forms. They can be intimate and long term or furtive and geared solely for pleasure with little or nothing said. Sexual cultures also vary within and among groups. Among the groups studied—primarily gay men, and heterosexual men and women—patterns differ widely.

Statistical studies reflect some of these variations. For example, in a systematic survey of sexual behavior in the United States, 67 percent of men and 75 percent of women reported they had had one sexual partner in the last year. Few—only 5 percent of men and 2 percent of women—had had more than five partners. For both men and women, race, education, or religion had little impact on patterns of behavior. Youths had more partners (among those 18 to 24 years of age, 9% had five or more partners). Overwhelmingly, marital or cohabiting relationships tended to be monogamous. More than 80 percent of women and 65 to 85 percent of men, regardless of age, reported no "outside" partners.[1]

Among gay men the story is very different. Although there are no systematic national data like those for heterosexual men and women, careful studies indicate that men who have sex with men tend to have larger numbers of partners. For example, a study using random digital dialing of 733 men (mean age, 40.5) in New York City who have sex with men found that in the past year, 47 percent had fewer than 3 male partners, 32 percent had 3 to 10 partners, and 21 percent had more than 10 partners.[2] Similarly, among those in long-term committed relationships, sexual encounters with others are not uncommon. Indeed, a careful review of what was known about gay couples concluded the "acceptance of sexual nonexclusivity is one of the most distinctive features of their relationships."[3]

Regardless of sexual orientation, sex takes on a wide range of meanings and functions. Men and women can use sex to dominate, exploit, humiliate, or express love and tenderness. Sex can also create openness and vulnerability. Within this spectrum, the sense of obligation between partners varies as well, shaping whether, how, and when men and women choose to reveal secrets. Few are completely trusting and truthful about everything. Some utterly lie or deceive.

However one thinks about secrecy, deception, lying, and truth telling, the possibility of transmitting a lethal disease gives these matters unparalleled significance. While questions of whether to disclose one's HIV infection to family and friends can produce psychological pain, whether to tell sexual partners can become a matter of life and death. The uninfected have to determine whether to believe a partner's claim of being uninfected or how to interpret a partner's silence.

Long-Term Partners: The Imperatives of Trust

For long-term partners, disclosure about HIV generally resulted from feelings of trust and security and the perception that a partner would expect the truth. The people we interviewed resembled those surveyed in earlier studies: men and women, heterosexual and gay, almost always told their long-term partners.[4] Yet our interviewees illuminated many critical aspects of the nature and dynamics of such trust that have been understudied. They commonly viewed trusting and being trustworthy as essential to the very nature of commitment. Trust seemed to be a basic drive, intensifying as the relationship developed.

Some experienced the sharing of intimate facts about their lives and the development of trust as a change in the self—an abandonment of the barriers that otherwise separate individuals. At the most extreme, a sense of merger could result. Larry, the HIV-positive New Zealander, said,

> There are moments when we are absolutely one being, there's just no distinction between he or me. And I think that's God, if you have to have it. That's God. But I think of it in terms of love. There's just such trust that you can say anything. There's no threat to our relationship about anything, anyway we think or whatever, and there's never been any sense of diminishing how we feel about each other.

Such trust could become the raison d'être of a relationship. Another gay man commented, "When a person becomes your lover, you assume that that means complete honesty, and that's the reason to be a lover." Such beliefs could be held even by individuals infected by those they had trusted. Maurice, a 46-year-old white gay teacher, thought he was infected by a lover who claimed not to have known about being positive. Maurice noted, "If you can't trust the person that you want to have a lover relationship with, then to me you're denying the whole purpose of having that kind of relationship." Women felt this impulse as well. Elise, a 51-year-old heterosexual Latina, an actress and a lawyer, who had been infected by a past lover, observed, "I wouldn't understand if somebody doesn't tell their partner. It's the person with whom you're sharing sex and intimacy."

Trust led to both truth telling and expectations of honesty, permitting individuals to tell their lovers about their being HIV infected and establishing expectations that those who were infected would reveal their status. Oscar, an uninfected gay man, asserted,

> I just expect somebody I'm being intimate with to be able to trust me enough to tell me the truth. Not just about that, but anything. If somebody thought they wouldn't be able to obtain what they wanted without lying to me, I would feel that that was really fucked up. I wouldn't really be interested in trusting that person and being close with that person again.

Trust could thus be a core element of love. Indeed, in the face of adversity, one woman defined love itself as "trust: caring for each other, being honest."

In relationships based on trust, mutual expectations—a sense of reciprocity—form a foundation of security. Sherri, the infected physician who felt that her professional survival necessitated secretiveness, said, "I don't want to be close to somebody physically who I can't really trust and who I can't be close to emotionally. I just feel like I need to protect myself, my whole self, more." Similarly, José, a 43-year-old heterosexual Latino who had been infected through drug use, said,

> I'm a man who feels I have a faithful wife. I have no fears of her whatever: she can go or do, or not do, whatever she feels like, and I don't have to worry

about anything. And if she's that faithful to me, why shouldn't I be that faithful to her? If she has something to say, she says it. And if I had to keep something from her, it would have to be something even worse than this, and how much worse than this can you get?

Many who viewed trust in this way automatically disclosed if infected and, when told of a partner's infection, provided support. Paul, an uninfected 31-year-old African American who worked for the subway system, had lived for five years with an infected man.

We grew close, and I guess once he felt close enough to me to trust me, he opened up and told me he was thinking about having an HIV test taken. I said, "OK, it's best that we have it done now, so there are no surprises." I couldn't go to the testing site with him on that particular day, but when I got home he told me he had something to tell me and that it came back positive. For a minute I was silent. It hit me hard because I wasn't expecting it to come back positive. I gave him a hug and told him, "Don't worry about it." We more or less sat down that night and discussed the future, and he told me he was scared, and I told him, "Don't worry about it, there's a lot of things out there that they can do to prevent this from spreading, so have a positive mind about it." I just more or less comforted him.

But even those who loved each other could fear disclosing, uncertain about how partners would respond. When Audrey, a 27-year-old white woman who was a Ph.D. candidate in sociology, found out she was infected, she thought about telling her boyfriend.

He knew I was getting the test result, so he had said, "Oh, call me," though he wasn't really concerned about it—but I guess enough to want to know what my results were. I guess there was a little anxiety. So I thought, if I don't call him, then he's going to think the worst, and if I do call, he's going to know the worst. I didn't know what to do. So I called him and told him. I don't remember his immediate words, but it certainly was shock and, "How can it be?" and that kind of stuff, and we arranged to meet on the same Metro North train going home. I got the train at the 125th Street station, and he got it at Grand Central. I was not functional. You'd think I'd got hit by a bus. So when we saw each other, he just held me. We were standing in the train. It was pretty crowded, and we didn't say anything going home, because I knew I couldn't. I would have lost it. When we got home, we just kind of crawled in bed, and I cried and he held me.

Though she feared rejection, her boyfriend, like almost all partners in intimate ongoing relationships, responded with support. She continued,

The big thing I remember from that half-hour or hour or whatever we spent laying there like that and him talking to me was how much he loved me. It really blew me away. It was just so powerful. I didn't expect it. I don't know what I expected, I had no expectations—but that just really blew me away. Six months after I found out, he proposed, and then we got married six months later.

Some sought to manage their anxiety by carefully staging the revelation. Nevertheless, impulsivity could overcome such plans. For example, Frank, a white heterosexual, was a former heroin user who had been drug free for four years and had attended law school for a period. He described telling his wife about his HIV test result.

I called her to tell her that I would pick her up after work, because I didn't want to tell her on the phone. I knew I wasn't going to tell her on the spot. I decided I would tell her personally. Well, I told her right in front of the office building where I picked her up. I couldn't wait, really. I don't even remember how much I thought about it, but as soon as she was in the car, I just blurted it out.

The emotional ties of the relationship and his need to share his burden had thus outweighed his plans.

Partners sometimes reacted with as much shock as the infected individual. Camille, infected by an earlier sexual partner, recalled telling her current partner.

I called him and told him he needed to come down to the hospital. He freaked out. He wanted an answer. I just told him to come. He arrived in a cab, dragging my daughter. His face was just really wild, he had money in one hand, my daughter's hand in the other. It was a cool day, but she wasn't dressed. You could see he had completely freaked and jumped in a cab. He couldn't handle any normal functions that were happening until he knew what was going on. They took my daughter to draw pictures, and we went in and the counselor said that I had something to tell him, and I just came right out and said that I had found out that my test came back positive. He was stunned. He just sat there.

News about a partner's HIV infection could impose strains on a relationship, of course, but having to confront such a threat could also deepen commitments. Jane, who got tested when she and her husband (who was uninfected) decided to have children, reported,

We used to fight, and I used to say to him, "Why don't you just leave, what is here for you now? You should just leave, go back to England, marry some-body and have the family you wanted. I can only drag you down." But I never seriously expected him to go and he never attempted to—I can't say he never considered it. There must have been times when he considered it.

Similarly, Paul, whose partner, Van, was infected, said, "He talks about, 'Well, supposing I get sick, are you going to leave me?' I say, 'No, I won't leave you, that's when you need me the most, and why would I leave your side?' I could never leave him like that. I can't even see how people would do something like that."

Deceptions and the Romantic Life

Although intimacy depends on trust and openness, complete and utter hon-esty rarely characterizes relationships. For good or bad, secrets, deceptions, and lies are often integral to romantic life. Such duplicity can subvert rela-tionships or make them endure.

Furtiveness may add to the excitement of sex. For example, like many other gay men, Morris, an uninfected white 42-year-old, harbored and even relished secrets about sexual encounters outside his primary relationship.

> My sex life was a big secret. I got a great thrill from the heightened secrecy—I'm doing something bad or wrong. It still plays a part in my sexuality today. I think pornography is a secret, a place to hide away and express something that you may not normally express to another person. Or sexual relations out-side of my relationship—outdoors, in a rest room or in Central Park, just get-ting a blow job here or there, fooling around at a urinal or something. I feel very guilty about it, that it's a deception, a lie—even though my boyfriend would probably condone it.

Partners also deceived each other about the seriousness of their commit-ment to each other. As Ernest, the screenwriter, said,

> In relationships, I've been deceptive—more in the sense of how serious is this relationship? I've stayed in relationships longer than I should have when I was afraid to be as honest—I knew my own mind but was afraid to state it. But I don't feel as though I'm someone who lies: like I was here when I was there, or I'll do this and then I don't. But I think I lie on the level of withholding in-formation sometimes, which is similar to this predicament. On one level is, "Do you love me?" "Yes," when maybe I don't. Or maybe I'm not sure. Or, "Are we going to be together?" And I'm not sure.

He thus distinguished between different types of lies and the moral valence of each.

Bisexual men now in primary relationships with female partners faced particular difficulties, placing in bold relief many of the conflicts and tensions involved. Jim, the computer programmer, had not told his wife details about his former gay sexual experiences or his current gay sexual fantasies. About the latter, he said, "It would serve no purpose to tell and would very likely cause damage." Then he went on to describe troubles he had encountered because of his honesty about past relationships with women.

> I made the mistake once. When you're first married, many times there's a curiosity about the lovers you've had in the past. I made the mistake of falling into the trap. She would ask, "Well, have you been with any other women before me?" And I said, "Yeah, I have." "Oh, what were they like?" And I made this stupid-ass mistake of telling her, even to the point of mentioning first names. To this day I can't mention the name Rita or Rachel or Susan without getting a sidelong glance and lots of jealousy. I don't see that mentioning a homosexual experiment by someone who was really just looking to find out who and what he was would enrich my marriage or my life. I could see that it would possibly be a great danger to what I consider to be a relationship—fairly fragile but becoming stable. Her difficulty with our marriage began well before HIV came into the picture, and HIV has only served to make it more confusing.

Of note, Jim switched to the third person in talking about his homosexual "experiment," not fully acknowledging his own sexual past. When asked if he ever lied to his wife, he responded, "Yes, it's kind of the rule," if the truth is "going to harm more than do good." He also did not tell her that he still occasionally went to topless bars and porno films. Here, he echoed David Nyberg's view that lies are justified if they protect or benefit another individual. The problem is, as Sissela Bok stressed, that such calculations may be viewed very differently by those who are deceived.

But despite the effort to use deception to strengthen or protect relationships, being found out commonly proved disruptive. Tony hadn't told his girlfriend about a recent gay sexual encounter or about his drinking. "She knows I'm bisexual. I had sex with one guy since I'd been with her, and I didn't tell her. I didn't feel really guilty about it either, although if I had sex with a woman, I would feel very guilty. It's kind of recreational and doesn't have any kind of emotional resonance." But he added, "I started to drink secretly, and then eventually she found out, about six months later, and she stayed around a couple more months, and then we split up and she left town."

Although deceptions and lies, from the blatant to the subtle, were not uncommon, most saw the issue of HIV as special because of the grave consequences of withholding the truth. As Ernest, the screenwriter, said,

> People find all sorts of gray areas when they're stumbling into that domain, whereas are you infected or not infected is pretty clear cut: that seems like a real lie of a different order, because of its potential consequences and because it's so black and white, whereas I guess the level of deceptions that I feel I practiced with partners of mine have been more like I've been lying to myself.

While most believed that their long-term commitments required disclosure of infection, some told only after recognizing that their diagnosis would otherwise be revealed by others—either those who morally condemned the failure to disclose or health care workers. Roger, a 50-year-old African American who had been infected through drug use, had ultimately told only his wife.

> It just came out. But I knew in the back of my mind that I was going to have to tell her eventually. I didn't want her to find out from somebody else: like I would go to the doctor and the doctor would tell her, or I come down with pneumonia and the hospital would tell her, so I knew I wanted to tell her in advance.

However, some did not disclose their infections to their long-term partners. These individuals failed to do so because they feared abandonment, or they did not feel obligated to be truthful or to protect their partners from the virus. Diane, a 44-year-old heterosexual African American who was uninfected, described poignantly what it was like to be lied to. She was stunned to learn that her husband had not told her he was infected, even while they continued to have sexual relations. For Diane, the "revelation," discovered as a result of her prying, nullified the premise of her marriage, providing a reason, perhaps a rationalization, for separation.

> I didn't know that he was infected. So I figured that if I wasn't infected then he wasn't infected, and no, we didn't practice safer sex. And then he didn't even tell me. I had to find it out in a diary he wrote. Everything just stopped. Everything. Lovemaking just went dead and I couldn't understand it. I figured that maybe he had somebody else. Until one day I was cleaning up the room—the other room where he normally be—and a book fell out. And being nosy, I opened it up and it fell right to the page, and it said, "I don't think my wife would understand that I was HIV positive." And that hurt me more than anything, and then when I asked him about it, he denied it. Because he said he figured I would reject him, and that hurt me very bad that he would even

think that way. I believe in my vows, "To death do us part, in sickness and in health." So we separated. Because he had no trust in me to tell me that he was infected. You have to have trust in a marriage.

A few men and women hesitated to tell long-term partners because of fears of ending a relationship that provided economic or other benefits. Though uninfected, Janet, a 43-year-old heterosexual African American, could understand why HIV-positive individuals would fear telling.

> Because they might lose the man. You hear people say, "So-and-so's woman got the virus." "What? That bitch got what? Well you better pack your stuff and leave. If that was me I would leave." Or you hear your man say, "Man, if that was me I'd get out of there." So then of course you're going to get scared.

Fears of rage and violence also molded decisions about disclosure. One woman, assaulted by her partner in the past, feared being beaten again. "When I was using crack I had to tell Jimmy, and I was scared to death. I thought he was going to grab me and I was going to have two more black eyes. But he took it well. Still, I was scared, scared to death." While this woman took the risk of disclosing, others did not. Wilma, the homeless woman, said about her partner, "He's a type of ignorant person, he's not educated enough. If he finds out I'm HIV, he'll kill me!" Similarly, Roxanne, a 58-year-old heterosexual African American who used drugs and was infected, feared that if she disclosed to one partner, he might try to hurt either her or her son. "I wouldn't tell him, because he's very emotional. He had a mania, and he might try to hurt my son. So why should I take the chance of telling him, and he'll think I gave it to him? He could have given it to me! I thought maybe he might try to kill me." In our study, those who feared such violence were most commonly women of color from poorer backgrounds, whose partners tended to be involved with drugs.

Thus, what would seem to be straightforward and psychologically and morally unambiguous—that partners in an ongoing intimate relationship would disclose their infection and recognize the necessity of doing so—turned out to be far more complex. While silence carried a price, so too did honesty. The potential toll of either disclosure or secrecy forced men and women to make profoundly difficult choices for themselves and others.

When to Disclose: Dating and Courting

The decision about *when* to reveal one's infection could prove especially difficult as well—particularly in the course of developing relationships. Uncertainty freighted decisions about the appropriate timing of such revelations.

Empirical studies of disclosure have repeatedly demonstrated that "new partners" were told less frequently than long-term partners.[5] A study in San Francisco, for example, found that one year after learning they were infected, only 50 percent had informed their new partners.[6]

Yet key questions remain. Should one tell about HIV when a relationship is just beginning or after a sense of mutual interest is established? Before, during, or after sex? In new relationships, particularly during dating or courting, a premature divulgence could end a promising union. Delayed disclosure could provoke cries of deception. Early on, disclosure might limit the pain of rejection. After a relationship has begun to deepen, rejection might be less likely but more injurious were it to occur. Beset by doubts and fears, plans to disclose could dissolve in the presence of a partner.

Given these potential difficulties, some chose to date only other HIV-infected individuals. Ginger, the former injecting-drug user who did not know whether she had been infected through sex or drug use, said, "I'm really not interested in going out with someone who's not positive. I finally made up my mind that I'd be much more comfortable in a relationship with someone who's HIV." For a parallel reason, Ben, a 45-year-old white gay man who had a history of depression and described himself as "almost a moral man," avoided dating younger men. He simply assumed that most older men were, like him, infected. "I pat myself on the back that I'm not in the situation of cruising guys in their twenties or even younger, because I don't know how I would handle that."

Occasionally, individuals did not need to tell a new partner, because the relationship had begun with an awareness of HIV infection. For example, Howard, the Philadelphia teacher, met his partner after speaking to an audience about being HIV positive. Social gatherings of HIV-infected individuals also protected against the anxieties of disclosure and the possibilities of rejection. Tony, the anthropology student who had been a cocaine user and sexually active with men and women, said,

> Someone suggested that Body Positive had a boat ride around New York. They said that everybody on the boat was positive, that it would be nice for everybody to meet someone, or talk, so it was open, there was no fear. I have a major fear with this: that if you meet somebody, eventually you're going to talk, it's going come up, and what their response is.

Similarly, Craig, the hairdresser and former male prostitute who always "played it safe" but found disclosure difficult, chose social activities that brought together infected people.

> I also play it safe by doing things that involve other people that are positive. Like Body Positive's T dance, for instance—that's a place where either the person is HIV friendly or is a member of the same club, so therefore it knocks down the responsibility of, "Listen I have something to tell you," and then having to deal with the response whether it be negative or positive.

Yet social events exclusively for HIV-positive individuals could also prompt ambivalent feelings. Craig recalled that he had at times avoided such occasions, "GMHC [Gay Men's Health Crisis] has a wonderful list of things for people to do. I don't participate in a lot. Not that I feel that I'm above it. I just don't feel comfortable in those situations or social gatherings. It just reconfirms the fact that you are positive."

But for those who did not have the security of attending gatherings of others who were infected, decisions about timing were inevitable. Delayed disclosure provided time for a relationship to develop and spared the pressure of telling on the first date. It also permitted one to keep HIV in the background psychologically, to maintain an image of oneself as healthy. Maria, the secretary who saw herself as a "private" person and a "goody two shoes," was direct but not immediate in disclosing to the men she dated.

> It's hard to decide when it's appropriate to tell them, because you don't want to scare them off and you also want them to be able to make the choice, and I've found it's better to let them make the choice. It scares them for a while. After I told one boyfriend he just wanted to take care of me and make sure I was okay, so we stayed together for the wrong reason. But he was also scared of getting very intimate, so then we broke it off.

Maria had also faced abrupt rejection from another boyfriend. She recalled, "It's just so painful sometimes to be rejected. I was cuddling with a boyfriend and told him before it got too close, and saw him backing off. That reaction left its mark." She told her current boyfriend after a few weeks.

> It was tough, because with this last break up that I had, I felt really bad about myself, and I wasn't even sure if I wanted a relationship. To tell someone when you're not sure about them is difficult. But I told him after three weeks. We hit it off. It was pretty unexpected. And I felt that in order to go on he might as well make the choice. And also, I'd rather get it done and over with because why spend all this time waiting, and then . . . It was early morning, and we were getting close or intimate and it was about the time that I should tell him, and I just get very upset when I tell them. When I tell them that it's something very serious, they just can't imagine. And when I do tell them they're really shocked, because by looking at me you wouldn't think that I was

positive. Because I work out and keep in shape, it's not what they think of someone who's positive. You can't beat around the bush; it takes me five minutes. I try to make sure I have the right tone: "What I'm about to tell you is extremely serious, please keep it confidential and do not speak to anybody about it," and then I tell them about it.

He cried, and held me. He was scared, scared for him and scared for me, because I think at that point we were realizing that we love each other, and we were just saying something good comes along and there's always kind of a string attached. And it's just a shock to them.

In the end, she believed she had chosen correctly. The relationship that she had feared might not survive the disclosure had "grown stronger"—supportive, but without the attention proffered by the earlier partner who had treated her as someone in need of "care."

While disclosure could thus deepen a developing relationship and enhance intimacy, the capacity to disclose often required trust that took time to evolve. As one woman said, "I cannot tell you something in a month when I don't know you that well. How could I tell you when I don't know you?" Speaking about a man she had known, she added,

I wouldn't have sex with him, because I didn't know him. To know a person, to really know their whole self, takes me around about five to six months or a year. You sit down, and a person wants to be with you and you want to be with that person, you want to talk your life to that person, and that person wants to talk his life to you, and you're really trying to know each other and their ways and they will try to know your ways, and that's how long it takes to find out about each other.

Personal divulgences and intimacy could also be mutually reinforcing. A single revelation could build trust that could then elicit other revelations. Conversely, lack of disclosure by one partner could perpetuate distrust. Only after a partner disclosed having a diagnosis of tuberculosis did Chuck, a gay African American who lived in a homeless shelter, disclose his own positive HIV status. "I said to myself that if he's honest enough to tell me he's got TB, I'm going to be honest enough to tell him that I got tested and I came out positive. That's how I told him."

Time and the emergence of trust thus led individuals to reveal their HIV status, but when the bonds of intimacy were far less intense, other motivations could prompt disclosures. Many believed that the risks of transmitting a lethal infection created a duty to disclose and a right to know, regardless of the type of sexual relationship. Others sought to avoid feelings of guilt. Basic moral impulses could thus inform these decisions. Disclosure before the first sexual encounter seemed logical. But what seemed appropriate in the abstract could nevertheless prove difficult. Ginger, who wanted her partners to decide for themselves what sexual behavior they felt was safe, recalled the anxiety that gripped her as she attempted to execute her planned announcement.

> There's a way to tell when the possibility of sex might be getting close, and I never tried to aim disclosure for that night. I aimed for prior to that night, and it would be something that I would have to work on for hours—how am I going to say this? It's probably the scariest thing that I've ever done in my life, to say to somebody that I'm dating and, like, "Oh, by the way . . . " I feel like I'm torturing myself: I got to tell him, I got to tell him, I got to tell him. I'm on a roller coaster and my stomach is in a knot and butterflies. Or I can wait until next time—because we're not going to have sex tonight—and let him really get to know who I am. I remember once we were driving around in a car and I thought to myself, all you have to do is say, "I have to talk to you about something." If you get that out, it'll be okay. And I just sat in the car, trying to get those words out: "I have to talk to you about something." And once I got that out I was able to be a little bit calmer and say, "Look, this is the situation, you know, I was tested, I'm HIV, this is what it means as far as a relationship is concerned." Nights have gone by where I've been out on a date and, "I'm going tell him tonight," and then I didn't tell him. But I just automatically know about myself that if I were to proceed to have sexual intimacy with him and didn't tell them, I would feel horrible for the rest of my life, whereas rejection wouldn't.

Her account reflects the drama and tension inherent as individuals weigh these competing motives, desires, and moral understandings, in trying to broach the subject. Like Ginger, one gay man was compelled to disclose so that he could face himself.

> If I was the top guy and was fucking men, I would tell them that I was HIV positive. I know that a lot of people don't do that in the gay world, but I would. And a lot of it has to do with wanting to be able to live with myself. I don't want to make myself feel bad by doing the wrong things. I want to be able to look people in the eyes and know that I'm okay.

Even when condoms were used and the risks of transmission minimal, disclosure could seem critical to avoid the shame of having to reveal the presence of HIV once the relationship had become deeper. Sherri, the physician who had told none of her professional colleagues that she was infected, said of those who did not disclose but practiced safer sex,

> I think that for some people it's okay to do that. I don't think it's a bad thing not to tell somebody, but I think it would be harder for me to go to somebody later on who I had sex with, even with a condom, and then tell them in retrospect. I don't have these little fly-by-night things. Even with the married man I was seeing, I thought it was going to be an affair, and I stayed three years with him! So I think it would be difficult for me to have sex with somebody, use a condom, and then a couple of months down the line, say, "By the way . . . ," or even just sort of lie, make it look like you just found out. I think that would create too much turmoil for me.

Thus, regardless of what might be morally permissible, some individuals held themselves to a more stringent standard of candor and felt a psychological need to be honest.

In a developing relationship in which sex had posed little risk of HIV transmission, revealing a new diagnosis of HIV infection could be eased. Emanuel, the former drug user, had not told his girlfriend he was going to be tested, because he had been unable to acknowledge—despite his history of drug use—that he could be infected. He had been drug free for two years when he learned of his diagnosis and had already begun to repair his life by entering college. He recalled,

> We were in a car, and it was dark. Night time. And I kind of worked my way up to it by telling her about having used drugs, and the connection between drug use and AIDS, and then being afraid to take the AIDS test for a long time, and then finally taking it several days ago and finding out that I have it. And then assuring her that the chances of her having it were minimal because I was using condoms with her ever since the beginning. That made it easier for me to tell her. If I had had unprotected sex with her, it would have been much more panic on both of our parts.

But in addition, he believed he could trust that his girlfriend would not reject him. "It was hard, but I guess I must have had a strong sense of her commitment and feeling toward me and our relationship for me to say anything to her. So although it was hard, in another sense I felt somewhat confident that she was not going to flip out or turn her back on me." Nevertheless, like others, he needed time to "work up to it," to make the disclosure.

Like Emanuel, others thought disclosure became necessary only as a new sexual relationship began to take on qualities of becoming more enduring.

Ben, the "almost moral man," recalled about a partner, "We were fucking each other with condoms, and I let him believe that I hadn't been tested for some time, and when I stopped seeing him as just a sexual being, I did get around to telling him that I had been tested." For some, disclosure at such a juncture was free of anxiety. Larry, the New Zealander, said, "I didn't tell him immediately, and I hadn't mentioned to him that I was going to get tested either. But as it became clear that we were going to commit, I had to tell him. And there was no trauma about it for either of us. It wasn't a big thing that I was leading up to. He knew to expect that I was positive." The strength of their emotional bond made the disclosure seem utterly safe. "I loved him, and I knew he loved me. There was just no question about it."

Yet plans to disclose before sex might be hard to carry out. George, the gay man who was studying for a doctorate in psychology, found it hard to tell his boyfriend when they began to date. Eventually he did, but only after they had already become lovers.

> When I met him, two weeks after I got to the city, I pretty much got it in my mind that we would take it slow and not have sex until I was ready to tell him, because I felt at the time that it seemed like a potential relationship. But it didn't work out that way. He seduced me—although I take responsibility for being seduced. But we found ourselves in bed kind of soon after we met. That was on my mind for the next month, and then finally it was very difficult to tell him. The primary thing was, would he reject me? And guilt and wondering how he would feel about the fact that I hadn't told him already. We'd been safe, but I didn't know how he would react. I knew I was going to tell him—just at a point when the relationship developed, where I felt there was some possibility of commitment there and some degree of closeness. He was wonderful. I'll never forget his response. He said, "You know, it's not that important" and "The color of your eyes makes more difference than that to me." Some of that was his denial, too, I think—that he was kind of minimizing it—but still it was very reassuring.

However, disclosure did not always have such a positive outcome. Dates could end when HIV infection was disclosed. Howard, for whom HIV was a central part of his identity, said,

> Early on after I first tested I had occasionally had dates, and over dinner I would tell them that I was positive. It was obvious it was going to be a sexual situation. It was heading that way. It was at dinner, and was obviously meant to be an all-night thing, breakfast included. Both of these guys I had known peripherally—we had circled around each other for a while before we actually

got to go on a date, so there was an indication that there might be a relationship developing. It wasn't a stab in the dark somewhere, in a dark hotel room or something. There was an indication that something could be developing, and I think that's part of it. If they thought they were going to have a relationship with me they needed to know who I was. And you could just tell the date ended right there. It didn't physically end there, but I knew that the date was over—that was it—through body language or the expression on their face or, "Oh my God, is *Roseanne* on now?" And I've seen these people subsequently and what was starting died at that moment. And I thought to myself, well, fuck that, who needs that? I was upset. I don't need to set myself up. And I'm not setting myself up like that anymore. I was putting myself out on a limb and got shot down.

Fear of such reactions informed much of the reluctance to disclose, and explains why often only a critical juncture in a relationship "forced" disclosure. Donna, a 44-year-old lesbian African American who had become infected through drug use, had been sexually involved with her girlfriend. Although the risks of transmission between women are very low, she had always been careful. But only when they decided to move in together did Donna share her secret.

I told her after I realized that she was someone who was important to me. I kept having appointments and was taking AZT, and we decided we were going to live together. I wasn't sick or ill or anything, but I didn't think that was something I'd be able to hide. Or even that I wanted to hide. So I told her. I tried not to think about it too much. I said better to do it now than later because I'd rather lose out now than lose out later. And so I told her, "There is something you should know. I was tested positive for HIV." And that's just how I said it. She said, "I thought maybe so because of how you were living when I met you, and we'll just be careful."

Finally, there were those who, despite a troubled conscience, disclosed only after moral promptings from others. Tony, the bisexual who had injected cocaine, would ultimately conclude that he had an obligation to inform his female but not his male partners. His sponsor at Alcoholics Anonymous made clear to him that sobriety required doing "the right thing."

I had dated someone just a few months previous to finding out, and when I found out, we had kind of split up. Then she called me. I said, "Why don't you come over?" And we were in my bedroom and began kissing, and we fucked and I pulled out when I came. And I felt really guilty. I wasn't afraid that I had infected her—I didn't come inside her, and I just didn't feel like I had really put her in danger. But I felt like I had really done a terrible thing by not giving her the option of deciding for herself. So the next day I called my sponsor and told him about it. My sponsor has been sober for many, many years, and he's very wise, and he emphasizes doing the right thing. And I felt that that kind of action was important to me to stay sober. Also, if I started doing bad things and keeping secrets, I don't think that I would be okay. My sponsor said, "Well, you understand what you have to do," and I said, "Yeah, I have to tell her." So I called her and asked her to meet me some place and I told her.

In short, in new and developing relationships, the timing of revelations proved difficult. As a result, some dated only individuals already known to be positive. Others delayed disclosing, permitting trust to develop and limiting the prospect of rejection. But moral intuition and convictions could dictate disclosure. For many, then, the desire to protect themselves from harm and the sense of moral obligation shaped the timing of disclosure. Most who knew they were infected traversed this complex conflict-ridden terrain. Far less common were those who either told immediately and readily or chose to remain silent.

What Is Told: Communicating in Code

People reveal secrets about themselves in many ways. Disclosure need not involve direct communication—for example, saying, "I have something to tell you"—but can be implicit or coded. By hint or sign, many sought to convey the possibility of infection in a way that avoided embarrassment and limited the humiliation and rejection that could result from more explicit declarations. A partner's response might then lead to further discussion or elucidation. But as individuals sought to "speak" indirectly, or without words, unclear signs had to be deciphered. Partners who understood that people with HIV could be secretive sought to "read" such communications. But it was not always easy. Thus, in the gray zone between deception—with all its attendant moral ambiguity—and truth telling, codes flourished.

Some thought HIV infection could be observed through physical, bodily signs. Tom, a 50-year-old white gay man—a former Catholic priest who had become a psychiatric social worker—was uninfected. He "watched for certain things—sometimes you see marks." Janet, when asked if she knew a partner's HIV status, answered, "No. But I know he's big and fat," suggesting that she believed that one could not be infected and look healthy. Carla, a 30-year-old lesbian African American who was uninfected, added, "I really couldn't tell you if she is or is not infected, because even if she does have it, she doesn't look like she has it." The potential ambiguity led another man to say about his partner, "His physical appearance looked quite healthy. But you still have to be curious."

The nature of "coded messages" ranged widely. Elise, the lawyer, recounted how one man told her that when she said she worked in AIDS education, "You were sending me coded messages." Some mentioned a medical problem, but not HIV per se. For example, Ben told partners, "I have a medical reason I should not be doing this." He went on to note that one partner responded, "'I know, I know.' I interpreted that as he was also HIV positive." Another gay man said about a partner, "During the course of our casual involvement, the facts of his lover's illness pretty much declared my partner's infection." Tom, the former priest, described a partner who sought to disclose in a guarded way. "He said something about weight loss, and I kind of followed up on it. Then he said, 'Well, I found out that I have leukemia.' I know he doesn't have leukemia. I'm sure it's HIV. He's really telling me that we aren't going to get together again, and he's letting me off easy, but he's also not going to advertise that he's HIV positive." Others said they were "negative, but that was a while ago." Paul reported that his infected lover, Van, had said to partners, "My results aren't back yet," rather than admit to being HIV positive.

Others commented more directly on their immune status—references that those familiar with the pathophysiology of HIV would understand. Craig, the former male prostitute, said, "Someone went so far as to say something about his T-cells. And once I picked up on it, I immediately let him know that everything was cool." He then went on to describe with great care his cautious approach to opening the way to self-disclosure.

> You sort of work your way around it. So if this person is willing to continue to see me, to date me, to screw me, and he knows that there's a possibility— nothing written in stone, but there's a possibility that I'm positive—that makes me feel a lot more comfortable and more than likely, somewhere along the line, able to tell the person. Because they're open, they're aware that there's a possibility, but yet there's no rejection. It opens the door to the rest. For example, at a club, the way I maneuver it is, "You ever been to the Body Positive T dances on a Sunday?" If they immediately respond, then you know that they've been there, are aware of it, or already positive. Boom. Another is just like a name or a place or anyone or anything that is affiliated with being HIV positive and you just slide it in there. Another way would be to mention I volunteer or have volunteered in the past with Body Positive or GMHC, and it opens a door a little bit, just slightly, and you feel a person out. You see how they respond. No one in their right mind is going to say, "Oh my God how

could you do that?" But you feel your way around it. It's awkward, it's scary, but it definitely has to be done.

Communication could also occur through a display of "evidence." Some left copies of *POZ*, a magazine directed toward the infected community, or bottles of medication visible in their homes, so, "At least the issue is out there." Gary, who was diagnosed in Queens at one of the first anonymous test sites, noted, "You walk into my apartment, and there are medicine bottles all over the place. I mean, it's not hard to figure out." Craig, discovering a medication in a sexual partner's living room, began a conversation he didn't dare have until then.

> I found an AZT tablet. It was the first time I noticed it. We had known each other for about six months or so, had been intimate, no unsafe sex no matter what the situation, but nonetheless I found the pill and I said, "Oh you take AZT." He says, "Yeah." I said, "How long?" He says, "Well about a few months now." The conversation was very casual. It's a very sensitive thing. You don't want to attack a person, or have him feel like his back is against a wall. So it just came out and we sat down and wound up spending the next twelve hours or so, as long as we could stay awake, talking and exchanging stories. But it wasn't brought up initially and definitely not verbally before sex.

A set of unwritten rules could shape coded conversations. When asked if he thought people told the truth, Van, who was infected and in a relationship with Paul, responded,

> When I was single, I said, well, if we use the rubber it'll be as if I told them. A lot of times, it would just not even be talked about. Some people would be bold enough to ask. But I would never ask. The best part about it, it was kind of like an unwritten rule: when you saw the condoms nothing had to be asked.

Although those who communicated in code usually believed they had met a moral obligation to disclose, others disagreed. Some saw such revelations as "half lies"—not as morally acceptable as the truth, but not as egregious as utter deception. Many who made such assessments understood the need to shade the truth. Tom said of the man who had told him that he had leukemia rather than acknowledging HIV infection, "It was a half lie. He probably didn't want to get it around that he was HIV positive." Yet Regina, who found out she was infected when her 7-year-old son was diagnosed, saw "half steps" as unacceptable deception. She said about a partner, "He's a good person, so I didn't want to half-step and play no kind of games with him. Half-step: when I should be coming out honestly with it, fully with it, I'm only half way. No matter what you may think about them, no one deserves for you to play with their lives like that." For some, half truths, half lies, and half steps represented adequate forms of disclosure. For others, failures to provide the "whole truth" entailed culpable deceptions.

In the face of uncertainty, many felt it necessary to probe. But as direct questioning could seem invasive, inappropriate, and difficult, inquiries about HIV often had to be indirect or coded. For those who were insistent on an answer, such indirection could abruptly yield to a straightforward challenge. Tom said about a partner,

> He came over, it was just going to be a half-hour visit and I had some vitamins and stuff, he had a bad fever. I think it was because he reminded me so much of my deceased lover John, I just asked him, I just said, "How did you get through the eighties?"—when they don't answer "I'm negative," I say "I've lost so many friends and it just seems to be a tough time." I'm waiting, fishing for an answer. When that didn't work—he kind of hedged on it in different ways—I finally just said, "Well what's your HIV status?" and he looked at me, and said, "I'm positive," and I just acted like it didn't phase me at all. But he never called me again, and I called him about a month and a half later, but I think he was so embarrassed, because earlier I could just tell that he really wanted us to be in a sexual relationship.

Finally, some were little concerned about the ambiguity of coded communications. Craig claimed that uncertainty about a partner's HIV status was in the end unimportant. He relied on nonverbal gestures to communicate intention to practice safer sex.

> If I meet someone in the club, and we like each other, you're hot, I'm hot, let's get together, we'll go to your place, my place, whatever, you don't talk about are you positive or are you not positive. What will come up, if anything, is, "I practice safe sex." Now that is a blatant statement that is not necessarily that I am positive, it's not letting you know that I'm not positive, it's letting you know that I'm not stupid. We don't exactly say it. It's not really a say. It's a do: a condom out on the table. You really don't discuss. Things just flow.

Silence and Lies

While some disclosed, if only in code, others remained silent or lied. Silence itself was taken by some as a kind of coded message, albeit one that could be especially difficult to interpret. For example, when confronted with silence, Tom took it as a signal. "One partner said he was negative right away. The other ones didn't say, which tells you something. Usually if you're negative the other person'll say, 'I am too.' If they don't say, 'I am too,' the chances are they either don't know or they're positive."

Yet more commonly, silence was viewed as an attempt at deception. Beatrice, a 41-year-old heterosexual African American who had traded sex for drugs and was uninfected, was angry that a sexual partner didn't tell her that he had HIV.

> One guy hadn't told me he's HIV. Even though we was messing. A friend told me. He said, "Well you know he got HIV/AIDS?" And I was, like, "What?" And this was a guy I was liking. He never said nothing to me. His friend said, "Didn't he tell you?" I had a feeling he had AIDS. He was losing weight, he had pneumonia a couple of times and everything. I had to tell him. It was at a moment where he was trying to be sexual with me. I said, "Listen, I can't right now because I'm afraid you have HIV. We been seeing each other, you romancing me and everything, and you haven't said anything. We're going to have sex and you wasn't going to tell me! I have to know, let me make the choice whether I want to play Russian roulette or not."

For some, silence was akin to lying—morally wrong, given the presumption that the truth would be told. The justification for Beatrice's anger was transparent to another woman. When asked if she could imagine not wanting to tell someone about her HIV infection, she said, "It's always like that in the beginning, but I also would feel guilty, or like there's something hanging over me, and I wouldn't be able to enjoy that person, because I knew it was kind of lying to them." However, others viewed silence less severely, as deception that was less offensive than false information. George, for example, said, "I'd rather not tell them I am infected than lie."

Silence could serve to hold back the truth, but others deceived more directly. Christopher, an infected 30-year-old white gay actor who had been a cocaine addict and hustler, said, "One time I was with somebody and he was pretty fucked up, we were both high and I could tell that he was sick after I really looked at him. And I asked him and he lied, but I knew that he was lying. But what could I say? I let him live his lie. I said, 'Are you sick?' He was like, 'I'm fine, I'm fine.'" Others provided suggestive but inaccurate information about test results. Although Craig did not claim he was uninfected, he did say his results were "inconclusive." "I've done that—not said that I was negative, but I have said that the test came back inconclusive, or once the test came out positive and the second time it came back negative, that all my tests came out—some bullshit—false positive or something like that. But that was when I was much younger also."

Many who gave inaccurate information distinguished between deceptions that left open the possibility that one was, in fact, infected and outright statements that one was negative. Explicit lies were more difficult to defend—viewed as morally more egregious. Aaron, a 55-year-old white gay artist who eventually went public about being infected through his art, said somewhat defensively, "At the beginning, I told somebody that I didn't know my status after I knew it. That was inaccurate. Or I hadn't been tested. That happened in the beginning. I've never told anybody I was negative." Similarly, Ben, who had described disclosing to a potential partner and then being rejected, had hinted at the possibility of being infected while asserting that he didn't know his status.

> I can think of a situation where I didn't give any clues and engaged in possibly less safe sex, and just have not responded or volunteered any information. And in a couple of situations I may have denied having been tested. Probably everyone that I've allowed to think I hadn't been tested is now aware that I have been and am positive. It was kind of a transitional step toward revealing my status. Since learning that I am infected I might say, "I guess I haven't done it because I don't want to know," rather than, "I haven't done it because there's no conceivable reason that I should." I may have expressed the belief that given my history of many partners over many years I didn't feel like facing the grim reality on paper.

The belief that such behavior was commonplace, almost normative in some settings, could make it seem more acceptable. Although he ultimately came to believe that sexual partners had a right to ask about his HIV infection, Van said, "If anybody tells you they're negative, I think they're a liar. First of all, if 98 percent of gay men aren't positive, it's a miracle, because I know about the lifestyle."

In sum, partners "read" each other, seeking verbal and nonverbal clues and physical signs, probing directly or in code. Some revealed only partial truths. Others remained silent, which some partners deciphered as evidence of infection. While some prevaricated, holding open the possibility that they were in fact infected, others lied more outrightly. Hence, partners might dance around the issue of HIV status in a complicated choreography, questioning each other only cautiously or indirectly; such silences or codes might or might not be interpreted correctly.

Why Not Tell?

Given the importance that many attached to trust in ongoing and even developing relationships, what could account for decisions to remain silent, deceive, or lie? Almost always, at the base of such decisions lay fears of rejection.

Rejection could occur even when unexpected, proving especially painful. The lesson learned would be hard to forget. Guadalupe, a 43-year-old heterosexual Latina who worked as a secretary, was diagnosed when she was 36. She told of a male friend who had expressed great interest in her.

> He kept calling me and he invited me out one day to dinner. And so we did go out to dinner, and somewhere in the back of my mind I had decided that I was going to tell him. But I was still uncertain and a little reluctant because of him being a cop. I felt that cops were hands-off when it came to people in my condition. We started talking, and one of the things he said to me was, "You know you're young, you're very attractive, you're by yourself. I don't understand why you have chosen to just remain alone. Is it because of your lover who got sick and died?" And I said, "Wait a minute, I think there is something that I need to explain to you," and I told him that my lover had died of AIDS, or I at least suspect that he died of AIDS. And I unfortunately am infected. "It's not that I don't want to see anybody, but this is a choice that I've made because of my condition." He was angry because, he said, "All these years that I've been talking to you, telling you my problems, this and that and you've never once said anything?" I took his kind of rejection to heart because here is someone that I was very attracted to, because I really did care about him a lot, I had very strong feeling for him, and before I had said to him that I was positive we had a conversation that was sort of like a joke, I think, and he said to me, "If I get divorced and ask you to marry me would you marry me?" We ended up taking the food back home, because I got very upset, my stomach got upset. And what happened was I never heard from him again. A week passed, two weeks, three weeks, four months, I didn't hear from him again.

Fears of disclosure could lead to indefinite delays or to promises to oneself to tell at a vague and uncertain time in the future. José, the former drug user, thus protected himself from the fact that he was dissimulating and argued that he was protecting his girlfriend psychologically, too.

> There was no way that I was not going to tell her. That never entered my mind. It's *how* to tell her, and the exact time to tell her, when it was more proper. I know I am infected, and I know she knows most likely I am, but how

should I drop it on her? So give me a day or two, it's not going to change. It wouldn't change if I'd wait months. But I was having the same behavior, which was doing nothing and just giving her a little more freedom where maybe she wouldn't have it on her mind, a few more days of ease, or not knowing, can't worry you.

But indefinite delays—however rationalized—carried a price, making it harder to disclose later on. As Claudio, the drug counselor and former drug user, recounted,

I didn't tell her in the beginning that I was positive, and we started having sex with the condom, and then there were a few times that we would be laying in bed and we started fooling around and the moment gets hot and we just start to go in and then I would stop to get the condom, and she'd say, "What you going to do that for?" And I'll get the condom anyway. Because I didn't tell her in the beginning, it was hard for me to tell her at the point when I did. I told her about two months afterwards. But I feel that if I told her in the beginning, and gotten it over with, it would have been much easier. I'm learning that either you're going to have to do it right up front and tell whoever it may be, particularly a sex partner, your status rather than to wait down the line, and then disclose. The way I felt was that all of a sudden it's like that trust thing comes in, like, why didn't you tell me earlier?

Because it might have led to exposure of a partner to HIV and betrayal of his or her trust, delayed disclosure could produce feelings of guilt. "I did feel bad. I felt guilty," said Charlene, a 44-year-old African-American drug user who was infected. "I felt like maybe I had trapped him, because we did have sex one time at the beginning without the condom, and maybe he felt that he should just stay with me now. That was the only regret I had—not telling him from the beginning."

Delayed disclosure could also produce enormous internal tension, burdening those with HIV infection as they endangered unprotected partners. Patrick, for example, who had planned to be a Green Beret, hid his bisexuality and HIV infection from his girlfriend and delayed telling her for two years. When he did disclose, he felt he had to lie about *when* he had been diagnosed.

We went out for a while. There's a real companion there, not just a one-night stand. Then she came over to my house. It was not going to lead into anything, it was going to be talk, have fun, then watch TV, and I was happy with the relationship going along that way. Maybe I knew her less than a month at that time. At that point she was very aggressive to me. I'm thinking this is going to take a few months. And it didn't take a few months, it was going to happen right now. And I did ask if she had any condoms, and at that point maybe my conscience was starting to work on me a little bit. She said, "No, we don't need them," and what happened then, I climaxed with her. It was very intense. And once it happened once, then it was going to happen again, because now I can't tell her. And it went on like that for a couple of years. I'm not proud of that.

So to me there was a lot of guilt behind it, but it wasn't enough to make me stop, because how am I going to tell her about a condom? There was a lot of guilt, a lot of fears on my part, because I thought she was still going to leave me. How am I going to do this? And it's going to fuck up everything in my life, but I had to tell her. For a year, I thought about it: how am I going to do it? I finally started to come to the conclusion that I'm going to lie to her. I'm going to tell her I just found out. I think it was going to kill me, holding it in.

Finally, one day I came out and told her that recently I went to a doctor and he said I tested positive for HIV. And I don't think we had done anything in the last week or two sexually. So I figured maybe it will make her feel that if we haven't done anything, she was safe. And I knew then that she'd also have to get tested. And she broke down crying, and it was very emotional. I guess we were there for an hour and a half or two hours, because she got very emotional. And then she turned to me and said, "Does that mean we're not going to get married?" I was shocked.

I expected her to leave me. And it didn't happen. And that still baffles me, and sometimes I've asked her, and she says, "Well, because I loved you, I really loved you." Maybe I didn't think she really did love me. I don't know, it's hard. Even now it's hard for me to bring that up, because I know that was wrong, I know that was fucking wrong.

I know people die with secrets, you see it in all the movies, they all have something. If there was anything in my life—and I probably thought about that a lot—that I was going to go to the grave with, this was going to be it. And maybe because my conscience started to work on me a bit. It said, you got to bring this out and take a chance. She's been tested four times. Each and every time it's been emotional. My fear is that if she did test positive, that I gave it to her, and I gave it to her in a more or less knowing way.

Yet his guilt was not enough to motivate him to reveal the truth. Fear that he would be abandoned was sufficient to serve as a countervailing force.

Ironically, fears of disclosure could keep two infected partners from revealing their HIV status to each other. Craig, the former prostitute who had known he was infected since late adolescence, recalled about a partner,

Before I found out that I was positive, and around six months after I found out, we continued to have unsafe sex big time, and I eventually told him. And it was weird because it was on my conscience, and it bothered me that I knew. He wanted the sex, it wasn't like only I did. But just the same, I didn't make him aware of my medical status, and when I did get the guts to tell him, he also told me that he was positive. Now, had we had this conversation in the beginning, we wouldn't have had to go through that.

Nonetheless, some delayed to the point of never disclosing, because it seemed too difficult. Rationalizations could be readily embraced. Ramon, for example, who had been drug free for ten years before learning he was infected, justified his failure to disclose both during and after relationships, since he felt healthy.

I've had two sexual partners and I didn't use any condoms, and that was a concern of mine. These partners actually never asked me about HIV. I felt that I was healthy because my T-cells were so high—about 1100—and I was given information that my HIV was inactive. I don't know what that means: it's in your system but inactive at the time. These partners didn't ask; I didn't say anything. I'd thought about it, I mean I felt kind of bad not revealing it, but then I said, if I revealed it, how are they gonna take it? I mean, we have a good relationship, we have a nice relationship, and as far as they know I'm okay. It's very difficult to reveal it. You want to deny it yourself. You live with a sense of denial, you want to be as normal as the next person.

Others searched widely and desperately for rationalizations—for example, seizing on unique aspects of a relationship to justify their decisions. When he first found out he was infected, Aaron, the gay artist, told his partner—and "sex shut down." Ultimately, he came to believe that it was politically important to make his infection public—through his art. Nevertheless, he did not tell one partner, justifying his decision with multiple reasons including cultural differences, but acknowledging that these explanations could be self-serving.

There's one person I haven't told. There's a language barrier, and actually I don't see him anymore—it's been about a year. I feel a little guilty about not telling him, but for me the relationship with him was kind of an escape, so I didn't. I met him at university. He was very protected. He lived with his parents, didn't have much experience with American men, and I think I just felt scared to tell him, basically. I was trying to protect him. He was Russian—I mean, a big cultural difference. I just felt there was so little I really understood about his culture. Maybe it was more in my mind a cultural barrier. I don't really know if in his mind it was so big. I feel I was just in a really needy place and I couldn't behave differently at that time, I didn't really know how to conduct myself.

Even in a relationship where one individual had revealed his or her infection, a partner might choose not to disclose, leaving the way open for assumptions—that may or may not be accurate—to be made. Neil, a 46-year-old white gay man who grew up in the South and worked in public relations, had long been closeted about being gay. With HIV as well, he generally sought the comfort of silence. Nevertheless, he told a partner in a new relationship right away, although the partner remained secretive.

I see more of him, and he knows I'm positive. He's never volunteered information about his status. I don't believe in asking people that information because they can always lie about it so what does it mean? I'm uncomfortable when people ask me, so I just assume that he's positive. His ex-lover died about a year and a half ago.

Finally, some acknowledged the morally troubling nature of their failure to disclose, but they nevertheless refused to change their behavior and divulge. Ramon, whose surprise at being diagnosed with HIV led him to be retested, had used condoms with his wife but not in two extramarital affairs, one of which extended over two years. Although he saw his behavior as "selfish," such awareness was not sufficient to alter his behavior. He could thus say, "These are very nice women, and I don't want to lose anything, any of our intimacy. So it was more of a selfish thing on my part. A sense of gratification. They were giving me a lot of gratification, and I said, 'Well if I tell them, it may put a damper on that.' Maybe not, but I just chose not to."

Casual and Anonymous Partners

The norms that governed the world of casual and anonymous sex differed markedly from those of ongoing long-term relationships, and even dating. Prior studies of disclosure showed that it was less common to reveal one's HIV infection to such partners than to those with whom one had a deeper commitment.[7] A study in Los Angeles, for example, found that self-disclosure was less likely as the number of sexual partners increased.[8] But why was this so? How did individuals justify their dangerous silence? Many gay men have "casual" sexual partners (often termed "fuck-buddies") with whom they have sex more than once, but with none of the commitments associated with an ongoing intimate relationship. In sex clubs, talk can crack the ambience; darkness fosters both mystery and fantasy. The rules and terms of these casual and anonymous relationships vary widely.

Craig, who early on had been less than forthright, described his current behavior as honest. "Anyone that I've slept with more than one time, I told." Yet others did not believe disclosure was necessary unless the possibility for a deeper involvement existed. Carl, a 41-year-old gay African-American masseur—currently living with his uninfected lover, Gerry, in an "open," non-monogamous relationship—remarked, "Occasionally, if I'm on the market for fuck-buddies or something, I will probably let it drop sometimes. I will mention it, if I think this is somebody I might like to see again, or if I think something interesting could come out of it." But where he felt no such prospect, he remained silent.

Typically with anonymous partners or one-night stands, HIV-positive individuals did not feel a need to disclose as long their sexual behavior posed little or no risk. George, the psychologist, spoke about men he had had sex with. "I met one person in a bar, one on the beach, and one at a retreat. Again, my feeling was always that as long as I felt like I was being safe, and I didn't feel like I really knew them, then I felt okay. I didn't tell them." Howard, the teacher, drew such distinctions as well. "If it looks like it's going toward a relationship kind of thing, it needs to be said, just because that's who you are. If it's a one-shot deal, it doesn't matter if you say it." Some sexual encounters, he suggested, did not involve his full self—who he "is."

In casual sexual encounters, secrecy could also be fostered by the realization that the odds of being discovered through ongoing contact were less likely. Karen, a 44-year-old African American who was infected not during her years of drug use but by her husband when they decided to forgo condoms, explained,

> If it's a one-night thing, I guess they probably figure as long as they're protecting their partner, why should they tell? But a relationship is different. The girl's going to find out sooner or later, especially if they're living together. It's going to be really hard for him to hide. I think probably he could do a good job, but sooner or later there'll be signs.

Moreover, in anonymous situations, talk could be viewed as anti-erotic. Of anonymous partners, Christopher, the actor and former hustler, said, "Usually they don't want to talk. Who wants to? We're doing it. The minute you talk about it, forget it."

For some, as noted earlier, it was as if truth and sexual pleasure were antithetical—disclosure could "kill the mood." Carl acknowledged that he occasionally had unprotected anal intercourse with his anonymous sexual partners and did not reveal his HIV infection. He, like many others, distinguished between the act of lying and the preservation of silence that hid

HIV infection. He would answer truthfully if asked, but otherwise he would-n't volunteer the information. But did such an outlook simply serve to jus-tify his silence?

> It kills any spontaneity. This guy I know tells people all the time when he goes out with them that he's HIV positive, and I don't. Now it's different if someone asks me. If someone asks me before we're to go home, "Are you HIV positive," I will say, "Yes." If someone's coming home with me for sex, obviously he's ra-tionalized to a point, I've rationalized to a point: he's protecting him, I'm pro-tecting me. Let's say for instance I'm into S&M and you're not, and we go home, and I say, "Okay, I'm ready to tie you up now, we're going to play with these needles," you're going to say, "No." So it doesn't matter whether I tell you or not. If you have the presence of mind to jump from a car that's coming toward you, duck or dodge a bullet, stop yourself from being tied up, you can certainly protect yourself from HIV. I was with someone once in a session who started quizzing me right in the middle about AIDS, and of course any interest in this person just died—completely uninteresting. It's like you're making love to someone and they start talking about dying. That kind of kills your passion, doesn't it? It's like kissing someone and suddenly you notice something hang-ing from their nose—immediately you're just not interested any more.

Indeed, an erotically charged mood could melt whatever moral qualms ex-isted. Christopher and his uninfected lover, for example, didn't discuss HIV with a third sexual partner and justified that decision by saying that this partner wouldn't have cared.

> I guess it's irresponsibility. It'll just ruin the whole thing, so you just don't. They do have a right to know. But it just was not brought up. In that moment, you don't want to destroy it. It's just fear of ruining the situation. But you know what? Most people don't care. I'm sure if I brought up, "I'm HIV," "Yeah, me too." Most people really don't care.

A moral obligation to inform—"they do have a right to know"—could thus be vitiated by assumptions about how little such revelation mattered to sex-ual partners.

Given the tacit norm against such discussion, many were surprised when the topic even arose. Lance, a 52-year-old white gay man in recovery from al-cohol and drug abuse—whose HIV infection was not diagnosed until he was hospitalized with AIDS-related conditions—reported, "I remember I was out one night, and I met this guy, and we were talking, and he seemed intelligent and he asked me if I was infected, and I was just really surprised."

Honesty about one's HIV infection could be even more unexpected. Sam, the respiratory therapist who had known his diagnosis for six years, recalled,

> I had met someone in a bar and we were talking and somehow we started talking about safe sex. I wasn't even really interested in going to bed with him or getting to know him better, and I don't remember who brought it up, if it was me or him. But he asked me if I was tested, and I said, "Yes," and then there was silence. I said, "Don't you want to know the results of the test?" And then I told him, and his response was, "Well, at least you're honest," and he walked away.

Such abrupt withdrawal could occur even after sexual contact had begun. Ben, who reported having denied to partners that he had been tested, said,

> Someone that I had become intensely involved with in foreplay at a bar became cool as ice when I felt the need to tell him. We'd been groping and licking each other's neck or something, and then I said, "By the way, I should tell you that I'm seropositive." I had the sensation of his fingertips getting cold and he removed himself very quickly from my space.

Rejection could thus take many forms, coded or direct, verbal or nonverbal, explicit or implicit. But whatever shape it took, in the end it caused pain and could prompt infected individuals to think twice about disclosing in the future.

Silence was not simply the choice of individuals. It could become a collective, mutually reinforced norm, with many engaging in an implicit policy of "don't ask, don't tell." In fact, at baths and sex clubs, anonymity and the absence of conversation defined the milieu. "It's just wham, bam, thank you ma'am," Gary, who now described himself as Mr. Safe Sex, reported. "So it's just very anonymous—that's part of the whole ambience." In speaking of the baths, Christopher, the actor, said, "At those things, people don't say, 'What's your status.' I think most people realize that no one's going to necessarily be honest. I mean, with these people you don't even necessarily know their name." Lance, who had been surprised when he was asked his HIV status by a partner, said about the lack of communication at baths, "It's just sort of unspoken. It's like 'don't mention the relatives.'"

Disclosure was as unlikely among those who exchanged sex for money or drugs as among those who engaged in anonymous encounters for sexual pleasure. Gloria, a 44-year-old heterosexual African American, had lived in a crack house and at one point had exchanged sex for drugs, but she used bleach to wash needles and was uninfected. She said, "I'm sure that there are quite a few that probably have just lied to get drugs for money." "Most people who have sex for money," a former drug user acknowledged, "don't say anything."

Remarkably, those who bought sex often seemed unconcerned about the possibility that sex workers might be infected. Dolores, who had not disclosed to anyone for two and a half years, said,

> Some people asked me if I had AIDS. I'd say, "No," and that's it. Some guys won't use protection. You got a lot of them out there that don't want to use it, and they know this thing is going around, so I'm like, well if you don't care, fifteen minutes of fun, and then a lifetime . . . come on, something's wrong.

As most men never asked or didn't seem to care, she felt freed of any obligation she might have had. Moreover, infected clients, sex workers believed, never disclosed, and some clients insisted that their sexual encounters occur without the use of condoms, paying a premium for their preference. Prostitutes had to adopt whatever measures they thought appropriate or possible. Typically, the women we interviewed took the risks necessary to get the money they needed.

Clearly, the subculture in which sexual exchanges occurred shaped the presence or absence and the content and expectations of communication, including disclosure of HIV. Some individuals assumed that their partners did not expect full or honest disclosure, legitimating nondisclosure—even when sex was unprotected—despite moral qualms.

Assessing Trustworthiness

Given these vagaries, assessing a partner's trustworthiness could prove difficult. Individuals drew on their own experience or training and sought clues in partners' character or behavior, gender, or the social milieu within which contact occurred. Often, psychological inclinations and characteristics of partners informed such assessments. The stakes were high, as misjudgments could lead to acquisition of a deadly virus.

The individuals we interviewed varied in how trusting they were. Oscar, an uninfected gay man, tended to accept his partners' revelations. "I think I would almost always trust them. I just expect somebody I'm being intimate with to be able to trust me enough to tell me the truth. I mean, not necessarily just about that, but about anything." But despite his trusting attitude, he acknowledged that at times people might not tell the truth. "It would depend on the situation. If somebody was groping me at a bar and telling me he was negative, I might not necessarily believe him."

Individuals drew on specific features or characteristics, whether physical, social, or behavioral, to judge the trustworthiness of a partner's disclosure. "Long-term lovers are honest," said Gerry, a 42-year-old white man, the uninfected partner of Carl, who was positive. "The short-term ones are mostly dishonest, I would think, mostly because of sex."

Some made assessments based on global qualities. Oliver, an uninfected 56-year-old white gay man from an old Louisiana family, believed that social class defined moral character. About a particular partner he said, "This is probably not a good way to determine these things, but if you're a certain class level and you come from the South—we're more a class society than they are here—you can tell. He sounded like he came from a good background, and I thought, well, he's a gentleman, I can trust him."

Others drew on a "psychic sense." Marvin, an uninfected gay African-American postal worker—who had never had an ongoing relationship, though he was 47—said,

> I use internal senses, what I call "psychic abilities," to perceive whether or not they're telling me the truth. So I'm not going to do this, that, or whatever. We can masturbate or whatever, but we're not going to get into serious physical contact. And those individuals where I decided I wasn't going to do that with, they're the ones who are dead.

He also gauged behaviors during dating. He had learned to trust those who spent time with him rather than those who rushed to have sex. While berating himself for a past lapse of judgment, he nevertheless drew lessons.

> With a guy who gave me crabs, there was momentary anger. There is a lot of self-anger that you let yourself in for something like that, because normally when you look at negative experiences of that nature, you pretty much saw it coming if you were sensitive at all. You could feel that there was something wrong. There's a certain kind of furtive activity or spurt that people place on you as to, "Let's do it now, let's hurry up and . . . let's go here . . . ," and the person who is in such a hurry is the one you'd better leave alone. The one who's willing to go to dinner, to the theater, to spend time getting to know you, pretty much those individuals are safe—the ones I spent time with—candlelight, wine, and song.

Yet such assessments, inevitably relying on ineffable qualities or uncertain or incomplete information, could be difficult to make. Otis, a 32-year-old white gay Catholic who trained as a social worker, had reason to be concerned, since he was not infected.

> If you're in a bar and you're not with friends, and you meet somebody and

start talking, you start making assessments. You can't know what's in somebody's head, whether it be HIV or physically violent acts. You can't see it, you can only trust it. So, one way or the other, you look at that person, talk with that person, see where their head is at, and are they a comfortable gay person? You sort of get general feelings, body language and whatnot, and from that you make decisions.

Many relied on "observation" to gauge trustworthiness. Janet, who had traded sex for money and drugs and who in years of prostitution, until 1993, almost never insisted that condoms be used, tried to assess partners. But she realized that she was ultimately taking a chance. Speaking of one of her clients, she said,

> In the beginning I remember asking him if he had HIV, and he said, "No." So I just take it as that. And then I caught myself trying to look him over, looking at this and to see, if they're undressing, if there's a lot of black and blue marks like the cancer that you get. Or on their tongues, see if they have thrush and stuff. But the disease could be at the beginning. So far I've been right, but I know you can't tell like that. So you got to take a chance and have the condom. It's not a game, but it's a chance kind of thing, too. You don't know what the hell to do.

Some relied on their professional training to provide guidance. Maurice, for example, drew on his teaching experience.

> Over a career of twenty years, you get to meet an awful lot of kids, and I just think that you get vibrations right away from somebody, whether or not they're being straightforward or honest or are covering something up. People can lie, and so on. But I have rarely been surprised when something didn't work out, because I sensed all along that there was something about it that wasn't really right. I wouldn't pick a person for a lover if I didn't think that I could trust them in more significant ways as well.

Gender often featured prominently in decisions about whether to view a partner as trustworthy. Gladys, the telephone company manager who had felt "numb" when diagnosed, had questioned her long-time lover about AIDS, but he had masked the fact that his illnesses were HIV related, claiming that his two previous hospitalizations for pneumonia were not for PCP. She asserted it was "very common" for men to lie. Similarly, Jane, infected by a former partner who did not know he was infected, said,

> I've never heard of a woman not either insisting on protection or telling her partner, whereas it doesn't seem completely uncommon to hear of a man

keeping silent or not using a condom, so I think it must be a little easier for a man to carry on having unprotected sex. My friend who died of it was gay, but he went on having unprotected sex for several months, at least, after he was diagnosed. Maybe it is for some reason slightly easier for men to do it. He never told me. One of our friends told me, so I never really had it out with him about it. I think one of my other friends did speak to him about it. He did eventually change his behavior.

Most troubling, and with potentially lethal implications, was that some saw men as less trustworthy but women as more trusting. Darryl, for example, whose life of drug use had resulted in years of imprisonment, said, "It seems like the woman is always more trusting than the man, especially if he opens up to her. That's what I heard from a couple of women: that they trusted men." But such views of men were not universal. Candor could be an expression of male bravado. Janet, who was not infected, said about her friend Jimmy,

I believe men are more truthful. 'Cause he'll talk about it to anybody, just like that. He'll see a friend of his he hasn't seen in years and say, "Yeah, man, I got the virus." I don't think I like him telling people that. I wouldn't say I didn't have it. But I don't think I'd just bring it up. But he will, in a minute.

She spoke about social rather than sexual situations, but was suggesting a more far-ranging point.

The social world within which people moved also shaped perceptions of disclosures about HIV. Within the gay world, some thought trust could be dangerous. Paradoxically, Oliver, the gay Louisianan who looked to social class to assess trustworthiness, was at the same time wary when describing veracity in sexual encounters.

I don't really trust anyone in the gay world when they say they're HIV negative. I think they're probably telling the truth if they say it, but I definitely know some who have told people lies just to have sex, and they were definitely not only positive, but two of them had AIDS. So if they'll lie about it— and they were nice guys I thought, too, till I heard that—then I had no more confidence in them at all.

About a particular past partner he added, "It's not a guaranteed thing he told me the truth."

Among those who lived in homeless shelters, doubts also persisted. Chuck reported, "It's hard to believe in a person that's telling you that he doesn't have it, because it's so popular, and people that come from the shelter, most of them have had sex with men. Because of the shelter. Not particularly because they're gay. It's like they go in the shower and start getting hot."

For those involved with illicit drugs, where crime, stealth, and harassment are common, trust could seem almost foreign. Gloria, for example, the drug user who lived in a crack house yet remained uninfected, said, "You can't trust nobody. If it was something that could be caught easily, somebody would do something to try for me to get it. That's how people are so cruel, you know. Nowadays, you can't trust nobody. Nobody."

Skepticism about disclosure could, on occasion, stem less from judgments about character and trustworthiness than from assessments about the inherent limitations of blood testing, which could, after all, determine only if one were infected at the time of testing. As Howard, the teacher, said,

> I don't trust anyone, not because they're lying, but because of the test. Somebody may know he's negative today. It doesn't mean he's negative tomorrow. It doesn't mean he's negative tonight, when you go to bed with him. That's just the way it is. The test could be outdated the week after they take it.

A few simply doubted the accuracy of HIV screening. Paul went so far as to say, albeit with rhetorical hyperbole, that he thought the test was "wrong 50 percent of the time." In the face of such objective uncertainty there was no alternative but to make judgments on one's own.

Given the enormity of what was at stake, searches for clues as to others' trustworthiness proved wide yet sometimes desperate or elusive—reminders of the difficulties of establishing trust more generally in an uncertain world.

Former Partners

Whereas disclosure to *current* sexual partners resulted from concerns about preventing disease transmission, maintaining intimacy, avoiding deception, and acquiring support, very different issues emerged when considering whether to notify *past* partners. Here, it was too late for disclosure to help protect against the possibility of transmission or to elicit emotional support. Thus, the decision not to notify was easier to justify. The elapse of time since the end of a relationship and the conditions under which the separation had occurred also hampered a sense of responsibility to warn of possible past HIV transmission. Indeed, a now classic 1990 study of gay men in New York found that 90 percent had not notified past sexual partners.[9] Yet how did our interviewees view and weigh these issues?

Belief that one's infection resulted from a past partner could provide a rationalization for not notifying that person. Tony, the bisexual former cocaine user, found the thought that he might have infected a past female partner "scary," even though his AA sponsor suggested that Tony might have been infected by this partner. Sherri, the infected physician, also wondered, "Maybe one of them may have given it to me. The last guy was very, very weird, and from time to time would say to me, like if he would get a cold or an episode of abdominal pain, 'I wonder if it's HIV,' like joking. But I think back on that from time to time, because he was just kind of reckless, he was a gambler, a nut."

One also could not expect from a past partner the support one might get from a current partner. In fact, in the absence of bonds of affection, former partners could well express anger and, if infected, retaliate. Ernest, the screenwriter who had received a letter from a former girlfriend that she was infected and who had known of his infection for less than a year, hadn't told all his former sexual partners, fearing their rage. "It wasn't so much feeling guilty, as reluctance to bring people bad news. If they were positive they would be very angry at me." He was also unsure how far back to go in notifying former partners. Ultimately he told three himself, and arranged for a fourth to be contacted through a public health department partner-notification program.

Remarkably, no one with whom we spoke had contacted former needle-sharing partners. As Emanuel, who had returned to college and trained as a social worker after becoming drug free, explained,

> First of all, I didn't know where people that I injected with were. To find these people I would have had to go into the jungles. And there was no sense of really having any direct responsibility, because once you're in a shooting gallery and you're cleaning out your works in a McDonald's cup, it's anybody's. So there was no real direct responsibility on my part. If I shared needles with somebody, they didn't necessarily get it from me. Sex is a lot different. It's more direct.

Although many did not inform those to whom they might have transmitted the virus, others believed both that a former sexual partner did have a right to know and that they bore responsibility for notification. A central concern was the potential medical benefits of disclosure. Emanuel, for example, was concerned not only about his former wife but about his son as well. "Why did I tell her? If I knew I had it, it was important for her to know—for herself as well as my son. We didn't use condoms, so I figured it was the right thing to tell her. Also, if she was positive, my son would have had to be tested. She went out and got tested. I mean, she said she did, and she tested negative." Ellen, the journalist who believed she had been infected through a blood transfusion, said, "I'd feel like I have to tell him because he might be infected. And if he might be and I'm the cause of this guy's demise, because he could have gotten treatment, I couldn't live with myself."

Disclosures could be made more difficult if individuals had had multiple partners, each of whom might react in an emotionally distressing way. Darryl, who had spent many years in jail on drug-related charges and was still adjusting to the news of his diagnosis, had a number of partners he might have infected. For him and others, such disclosures represented a journey— a process with stages, each shaping the next. In the months since learning he was infected, he told some, but not all, depending in part on whom he happened to see.

> The hardest thing to do is to tell somebody I'm HIV positive, and they might be and have to get tested. My fiancé has a few friends that she's very close with, and she shared it with one of them, who shared it with a boyfriend, who is real good friends with one of my ex's with whom I had my son. And this boyfriend went back and told my ex. The first time my ex asked me about it, I lied and told her, "No." But I finally admitted it to her. I had a lot of fear—more for selfish reasons. Even though there was some concern, it was more about what she'd probably say to me and things she'd call me, and she might not want me to see my son again—a whole bunch of stuff. And when I told her, none of those things came to pass.
>
> Plus she has a right to know. Because I believe she could at least have a choice in how she chooses to take care of herself better. It was scary telling her. The biggest fear telling someone is what their reaction will be. Will they automatically stop loving me, caring? First when I told her, she got quiet on the telephone. Then she asked me how long I knew and I told her and she asked me why I did not tell her when I first found out. I told her I didn't know how.
>
> After she had found out, I felt a relief, and I called another friend and told her that maybe she should get tested because I'm HIV positive. And she did, and she's positive. She was never an IV user but she used drugs years ago. And just Thursday another young lady came to me and asked me. She said she had heard I was HIV positive. And by that time I had already shared it openly, I had told just about everybody. It's real stressful worrying about who knows and who doesn't know, so she asked me and I told her. She started crying, and talking about her daughters and she wanted to see them grow up and graduate, and she also shared with me, too, which most of them did: why didn't I tell them as soon as I found out? Later she told me the test was positive, and she started crying, saying her life was over, she was going to die. I listened and let her go through it. I gave her the number to the support group, and she went. I think she's doing all right. But I do feel guilty.

I believe it's important to come to some level of acceptance with it and then, if you can, let the other person know. I guess I feel that way, because I constantly remind myself that had it been the other way around, I believe I would like to know, I really would.

Here as elsewhere, individuals invoked the Golden Rule as a motive for moral behavior.

Despite the sense of duty, some chose to notify particular kinds of partners but not others. Jim, the computer programmer, now married, had had a number of homosexual "experiments." He decided to contact the women, but not the men, with whom he had had sex. "The men I couldn't find because I don't even remember their names at this point." Moreover, he assumed that the men had greater reasons to suspect they were at risk and could seek testing on their own. He revealed as well the difficulties of acting on these decisions.

When I found out, my first reaction was of course to protect my family, but the second one was to call lovers that I've had before and check on them. And the only one that I have not been able to get in touch with, except for the men, is Rachael. I felt it was my duty to warn them to be tested, and if they could profit from the knowledge in their own continuing sex lives, then great, I'm doing them at least one service, regardless of any hurts or emptiness of the past. A month after finding out about myself, I began to try and track them down, and it took me the next eight months to run down those seven women.

I could picture all kinds of husbands and boyfriends hunting me down to kill me if, God forbid, one of the women should be infected themselves. Also at the time I didn't expect to live very much longer anyway, so to me it was perhaps fear of violence rather than fear of death or fear of ostracism or any of that. It also took a long time because I couldn't do this openly at work. I couldn't call people and talk to them over the phone about this. At home I couldn't do it either, because at the time my wife was insanely jealous, shocked, and then fearful for herself. She didn't know that I was doing this until very near the end of it. She was very angry that I did this. Because she felt that I was getting in touch with these women for romantic reasons, or that they were on their own and deserved what they got. Finally, after about a month of sitting and thinking about it and helping me track down the last woman, she decided that it was perhaps the best thing to do, but I shouldn't try too hard. She allowed me to do it from home. The last woman that I was trying to track was Rachel, so I was trying to work the connection through calling from home instead of pay phones.

I feel that it was a duty to tell them. It's a personal responsibility that every-body must shoulder for themselves, and if they refuse to, then something else has to step up to the plate, some other agency or entity. I asked the women, "Can I call you in about two months so that you can get your test and get your results back?" They were all negative, and very happy at the end, and very thankful to me that I did take this time out.

Other logistical difficulties arose in trying to locate former partners. Nancy, a 32-year-old white heterosexual, a former textile designer, learned she had HIV during a hospitalization for PCP. She noted, "People move, especially in their twenties. I was going to college, they're going to college, phone numbers and things move. It's not like you have the same house for twenty years, so that's a hard part."

But clearly, not just logistical problems had to be confronted. When part-ners had separated in anger or on bad terms, reestablishing contact was all the more difficult. Nancy added, "It's not always easy to talk to an old lover, because why did you break up? I mean, there are problems there. Something that's not right, a lot of times anyway." Whereas some, as we have seen, took this as reason enough not to try, many believed they had a duty to reach out to former partners, and they saw this issue as but one among others in mak-ing a decision. Keith, who worked for the phone company, recalled about one partner, "We had a bad falling out, and broke up, and just recently started somewhat communicating, and were able to tolerate each other's company, because we have all the same friends. Now we're sort of going to the same events. But there hasn't been an open line of communication." He was able to inform his former girlfriend—once they had reestablished a con-text within which to talk—but not his former wife, with whom he had shared a life of drug use. He felt no need to contact or inform her.

> She was my drug partner, and I don't live and behave in the same ways. She is still involved with drugs. And I just found out a few days ago that my 15-year-old daughter is pregnant. They're still locked in that world, and to me it's a world of continuous depression, and you don't know till you come out of it, hey, God, I'm not there anymore. So communication with her is impossible. I don't know how I did seventeen years with this woman. We went from the drug addiction arena, me coming out of it, almost a near eviction, and zero money, to me now being able to enjoy some things and build my life back up, and she has absolutely no respect for that.

Indeed, his comment that he "did seventeen years" with her reveals that he had experienced his relationship almost as a prison sentence.

Some who endorsed, in principle, the importance of notifying former partners could forgive individuals for not doing so, given the difficulties involved. Moral, psychological, and logistical issues got weighed against each other. Ellen, the journalist who just three months earlier had learned she was infected through a blood transfusion, reported, "If somebody called me and said that they had it, and I had sex with them, they might have prompted me to get tested because it's really hitting home now—so-and-so's got it. I guess I would have wanted him to notify me, but I don't think I would have felt bad if he didn't. I couldn't blame him if he didn't." For herself, she didn't know how she could even begin the task of locating her former partners.

> I thought about it, and first of all I don't know beyond being a super-sleuth and really making this my calling, it would be very hard for me to do because a lot of the people I lost touch with. They were people in college and from different areas. There's one person, if I think about it, if I was to tell anyone—we realized we were better off being friends and once in a while we talk—but I know he had sex with ten million other women, and who's to say I gave it to him?

Although many former partners who were contacted were grateful, and none retaliated, some infected individuals nevertheless found the process of notification too difficult and emotionally charged to undertake directly, and they sought other modes of anonymous communication. Sherri, for example, the infected physician who sought to protect her own confidentiality, sent unsigned letters.

> I wasn't in touch with my previous sexual partners, and I really wanted to tell them, especially since I thought I might have gotten it as early as '84, and I really was very concerned. I wrote them letters. I did it on a PC, and I don't know how I managed to get their addresses even though I wasn't in touch with them. I mailed the letters from Newark, New Jersey, and I wrote this letter seriously, because I didn't want it to seem like a joke, like a chain letter or something: "You have been exposed to HIV, and you may have been infected and this is not a joke." I sent three letters. One of the men had previously worked at the hospital where I worked and I knew that a year before he was living in Illinois. So I got a person that I worked with to look at his file and give me the address. For the other one, I just had his address from before, and I had assumed, since I didn't hear anything, that he hadn't moved. The third one, interestingly, was the most difficult and the one I was involved with most recently. I hadn't spoken with him for about a year before I found out. But he

was a married man, and I couldn't send it to his home, and actually I don't even think I had his address, but I thought it was the most important that I tell him. So I sent it to his work. But I put an envelope in an envelope in an envelope, and I wrote "personal, confidential," all this kind of thing, and I sent it to his work. I had the address.

There were two earlier men. Mostly, I don't know how to get in touch with them, that was the main thing. And questions of whether I could have given it to them, that was also my concern. One of them was impossible—he was my first sexual partner. So one of them wasn't even an issue, and the other one I really had no way of getting in touch with.

Those who found any direct involvement in the notification of past partners too difficult had the option of using partner-notification programs established by local health departments. Yet some found such programs threatening, wary that their own privacy interests would not be protected. As a result, when approached as part of a health department–initiated effort, a few provided inaccurate information. For example, Donald, the uninfected closeted bisexual who was tested while in prison, once lied in a partner-notification effort for syphilis.

Back when I was in the group home I caught syphilis, and when I went to the hospital they gave me some pills for it and asked me how I got it, and I said my partner, my friend, because there was only one partner or person I was with. They wanted me to reveal who the person was, and I couldn't really do that because I didn't feel right. But I did go back and confront that person. I told the doctor it was a girl, but it wasn't a girl. I was in a home, and I didn't want people to find out. Whatever happens, the counselor's going to tell people at the home, and I didn't want them to find that I was gay, so I just let it slide.

Such fear-engendered dissimulation may limit the full effectiveness of partner-notification efforts.

Others, however, saw public partner-notification efforts as useful. Patrick, the closeted bisexual police officer who had wanted to be a Green Beret, used such a program to contact three of his four past female partners. He himself notified the woman with whom he felt a closer bond.

I did partner notification. I knew it had to be done. I started hearing about people doing it, just in general in AA. And I thought maybe I should do this too. Maybe I should step out and tell these people. There was a Department of Health unit that would do it, and I did that with the three girls after finding out. The other girl, from '83, '84, was more of a personal friend. The three I didn't know well enough. I wouldn't stand out in their mind, and maybe it was easier.

Although he had turned to a public agency, he thought the route of personal notification was more desirable.

> I would rather be told by somebody more personally than somebody that has had no contact—just two people out of the fucking blue who walk up to you, and say, "We're from the Department of Health." So I said if I could do it with her, and it goes easy, then I'll go with the others. But it didn't go that easy with her. I realized I can't fucking do this with the others. The other ones I did not know that well. Maybe that's cold and callous, and maybe it made it easier for me. I just didn't feel I could actually hold up any more. So I went to the Department of Health and gave them what I did know about the other girls.

Partner-notification programs seemed especially useful for those who wanted a former partner notified but feared how the partner might respond and how their own reputation could be affected. Nancy, the former textile designer, used such a program for a former partner from a small community. "It's too small of a town. He could be a real bastard about it. It's just too small of a place and I go back there."

But not everyone thought such public health programs satisfactory. It is noteworthy that Sherri, the infected physician, found the New York State partner-notification program bureaucratically inadequate. "New York State has this thing, and I tried to look into that, but I came up with actually a lot of difficulty. I wanted to tell them that I was a physician treating a person I might have placed at risk, and I just got a lot of bureaucratic red tape."

Those who felt morally obligated and braved their own fears about contacting past sexual partners—especially ones who had no reason to suspect being at risk—could not understand others' failure to use such privacy-preserving approaches as anonymous letters or public health partner-notification services. Jane, infected during an affair with a man who did not know he was infected, spoke of such a situation.

> I have a very good male friend who has a son, and the mother of the child and the child, who is about 8, now live down South, and my friend lives up here and is not exactly sure how long he's been infected. So it's conceivable that both the mother and the child are infected. He hasn't told them about himself, so I suggested that he have an anonymous letter sent so she could at least get tested. In that way, if he's uncomfortable signing it himself, it would have

the same effect, and he would be kept out of it. I don't believe he has done anything about it, and I do think it's morally wrong.

Strikingly, those we interviewed, while commonly confronting the issue of contacting former sexual partners, did not recall physicians or counselors ever raising the topic, although sponsors in AA and some family members did broach the topic. Nancy, who believed that unsuspecting past partners had a right to know, recounted, "Nobody has directed me in the right place for that or helped giving me any kind of guidance on that. That's been completely ignored."

The notification of past partners thus tested the limits of obligation to those one might have exposed to HIV. The bonds that mandated such disclosure in ongoing relationships did not exist. Prior bonds usually eroded when ties ended. The past was past. Moreover, there was now no possibility of offering protection. Most of the men and women with whom we spoke struggled with this issue. While some concluded that the burdens associated with disclosure outweighed the potential benefits, others nonetheless felt duty-bound to notify those they might have endangered.

In contexts as vastly different as ongoing loving relationships and fleeting, furtive sex, issues such as truthfulness, prevarication, and silence—resulting in either dissimulation or outright lying—challenge conventional assumptions about the moral worlds we inhabit. Although Sissela Bok and David Nyberg disagreed about the primacy of truth telling, they concurred about deceptions and lying that placed others at risk. Indeed, in the universe occupied by moral analysts, few would defend the silences, deceptions, and lies of many of our interviewees. This gulf between the realms of moral judgment and everyday life could not seem starker. Yet this chasm invites us to probe the wellsprings of these decisions made in the face of basic needs and terrible fears. Our analysis does not preclude judgment, but it calls for a moral sensibility informed by an appreciation of the conditions under which these most vulnerable individuals were compelled to act.

3 | SECRETS AND "SECRET SECRETS"

Disclosure in Families

With parents, children, sisters, and brothers—relationships in which transmission of HIV is not a risk—disclosure poses very different challenges than with sexual partners. How did infected men and women feel about revealing their diagnosis to family members other than their spouses? What did it mean to do so? After disclosure, what did infected individuals expect or feel they had a right to expect from kin, in terms of emotional support and maintenance of confidentiality—crucial for people living with the virus?

Family relationships range enormously in levels of candor and openness, depending on the topic in question: speaking of hopes, aspirations, disappointments, and sorrows differs dramatically from talking about sex and physical desire. Specific family histories, filled with love and anger, shattered or fulfilled expectations, support, conflict, and competitiveness, shaped how much individuals felt safe or needed to reveal themselves. The emotional styles of families also informed rules of disclosure. Families vary in style from open and expressive to more restrained patterns of interaction. As Carl, the gay masseur, said, "We're not a gush family. We'll tell each other we love each other at the end of our phone conversations, but that's about as deep as it goes."

The complexities of family dynamics could well lead to avoidance of a matter as serious as HIV infection. Such dynamics could fashion explicit rules of revelation. As one woman said, "In our family there are secrets, and there are 'secret secrets.' A secret is something everybody knows but agrees not to talk about. A 'secret secret' is something nobody knows." But what does it mean to know but not broach a secret?

Family members often spoke of obligations to each other—particularly parents to children, adult children to elderly parents, and sisters and brothers to each other. Bound by those responsibilities, they had to consider whether disclosure could represent a kind of "thoughtless honesty," more injurious than helpful, or whether the failure to share the truth would be experienced as a painful withholding, a rejection, a failure to meet legitimate expectations.

Telling Parents

Many found disclosing to their parents one of the most difficult but unavoidable tasks they faced. Earlier studies showed that individuals find it easier to tell their mothers than their fathers.[1] But confronting either parent is still hard. Closeted about his bisexuality, Peter, an infected 31-year-old white physician who was married, felt he had no option.

> It took about three months after I found out before I decided to tell them—just a matter of finding the right time, not that there ever is a right time to tell somebody. It was difficult, but I felt it was something I had to do. I know that they could tell something was wrong, that something was going on, in the way I was acting.

When, if ever, is the "right time," given that most adults do not now live with their parents and interact with them primarily on specific occasions or on short visits?

Given the nature of familial expectations, many felt that disclosure was necessary and would generate support. George, the psychologist, thus turned to his mother and siblings.

> I told my family right away. It was very, very hard, but it wasn't an issue of whether or not my family would be accepting. If anything, it brought me closer to everybody in my life. But what is the alternative? To not tell? How could I be at all close with anybody and not let them know? Plus, it's not fair to them, and it really deprives me of the potential support that I get from the relationship.

After being diagnosed with HIV, many did turn to parents first and foremost. Regina, when learning that her son, Timothy, had AIDS and that she too was infected, turned to her "mommy." Like others, she found that doing so lifted the burden of isolation.

> My mother's baby sister raised me, so I call her "mommy." She was the first one to know anything about it. I needed someone I could share with. I felt shame, shame, utter shame, that my lifestyle was now taking Timothy's life. I couldn't look in her face. I could tell she was hurt. She was afraid for me, afraid for what the baby might be going through. But she didn't make me feel alone. I knew that someone was there for me. She was very, very kind about it, very kind.

But not all adults were close to their parents, and serious obstacles could exist. For example, a past history of having disappointed parents could create problems and make disclosure more difficult. With many years of imprisonment and drug use behind him, Darryl feared that telling his mother would injure her yet again. "I remember when I was about to tell her, I was thinking, damn, I did so many things to hurt her, do I need to tell her something else that's really gonna hurt her? And I told her, and she started crying, like I shouldn't have told her. But I did it. She's very supportive."

The desire to be open could conflict with concerns about burdening parents. Indeed, surveys have found that the desire to protect one's parents is what makes such revelations so difficult.[2] But how did individuals struggle with these opposing moral virtues: telling the truth versus protecting the vulnerable? Another drug user, Dolores—the "black sheep" of her family and former street hustler, who disclosed to no one for two and a half years—feared that candor would hasten her mother's death. Yet, in the end, the act of eventually telling her mother and encountering her mother's dismay motivated Dolores to detoxify from heroin.

> My mother was really sick. I didn't want to let her die, lying to her, but I didn't want her to worry. I'm the only one that's ever been on the street, and she always worried about me. I figured if I told my mother I got AIDS, this was going to kill her quicker, because she is going to be worried to death about where her child is, is she alive? I went over there to eat, because I come over when I want. My mother always gives me a couple of dollars. So we were just sitting in the room talking. She said, "You look like you're losing weight, like you're sick or something." I said, "Why do you say that?" "Because you don't look like that." "Oh Ma, you only trying to make somebody sick or something," I said. "Oh man, Ma, I can't hide it no more, I got AIDS," "You got what? How do you know?" "I got it, Ma!" "I know God was going to take you out of here," and that's how it went. She be worrying about me if I don't do the right thing. Then I got to get myself together, and that's when I went into detox.

The act of disclosure could thus make the diagnosis more concrete, forcing individuals to confront it more fully themselves.

Parents could surprise their children, responding with acceptance when dismay or rejection was anticipated. Christopher, the gay actor, was torn about disclosing to his mother, who reacted in an unexpected way.

> She's been through so much in her life. My brother was killed and my father died, and then I was sick as a kid, and then my sister went through a drug-ad-

dict stage and was in rehab after rehab. I thought, this poor woman has been through so much that I did not want to tell her, because I don't think she would have been able to understand it, know that someone can live and be healthy and still be HIV positive. So it was hard for me to tell her. But I finally did. Now my mom is Miss AIDS, buying books about it.

Although many parents demonstrated unexpected levels of concern and support, others' reactions to an offspring's infection mirrored the troubled nature of the relationship before the disclosure. For Tony, bisexual and a former cocaine user, his parents' reaction resembled their response to his years of drug use.

I called before Christmas. My stepfather answered the phone. And I told him. His first reaction was, "How do you think you got it?" Meaning, are you telling me that you're gay. I said it was from shooting drugs. We talked about how to tell my mother. When she got home he would sit her down and tell her and they would call me. So he did that, they called, and my mother was very closed down and seemed angry at me.

A poor response could come as a surprise, making it all the more painful. Chuck, the gay man who lived in a shelter, turned to his mother, from whom, he said, he kept nothing. He felt unburdened, but also stung by her fear, which he experienced as rejection.

Me and my mother are very close. So I told her right away. I went over to visit her because my brother just had died from, I believe, the virus. I felt better about it because I wasn't hiding nothing from her. She asked me to use certain dishes in the house—like if I wanted some Kool-Aid or a sandwich or something. I was disappointed. I was thinking, but damn I'm still your son. It seemed like I was pushed away from the love that she had for me when I was a child—saying that these are your separate dishes to use. I still kiss my mother on the cheek all the time when I come and go.

Fear born of ignorance about how HIV can be transmitted could thus be experienced as stigmatizing and degrading.

Among the concerns expressed by our interviewees was the extent to which parents could be trusted to maintain confidentiality. Strong expectations led to intense disappointments when parents told others. Sherri, the physician, said,

I was very upset. More than upset, especially because, of all the people that I really felt that I could trust—in fact when I told my mother she said something like, "Well I would never do anything to hurt you, I will never tell anybody, I will hold this in the utmost." She was the last person that I expected to say anything. So I was just very hurt. But at the same time I understood it because I understood the circumstances in which it happened. My sister who had been living in Maine came into New York for the weekend, and my mother was still in her adjusting period, and broke down and started crying over dinner, and then it just kind of came out. So I understand, I could just picture it happening. But at the same time it made me more cautious to tell anybody else.

Sherri here placed in bold relief the tension between a child's need for privacy and a parent's own need for support in the initial period of grief—a need that could prompt sharing the diagnosis with others.

Occasionally, individuals planned to disclose eventually but hesitated for a variety of reasons, such as waiting for clarification of diagnostic issues. Jim, the married computer programmer infected through earlier gay "experimentation," waited to disclose to his parents until it was clear that neither his wife nor his two children were infected.

I could easily tell them. I could go to my mother on the way home from Jersey and say, "Mom, I'm HIV positive, I don't know about the kids. I don't know about my wife. We'll let you know," and then see her suffer for the next six months. So I said to myself, I'll wait until my wife's second test, which I did. I told them all, because they're important in my life. And that means that you share your joys and your sorrows.

In defining the importance of family as sharing both good and bad news, leading to celebration or support, Jim emphasized a theme of continuity and wholeness. Within such a family, disclosure to parents seemed natural; the failure to disclose, a violation of expectations.

Others waited until they felt emotionally prepared to provide the support that family members, shattered by the news, might demand. Audrey, the Ph.D. candidate in sociology, learned in her early twenties that she was infected. Based on her parents' past responses to bad news, she knew she would need to be strong when she told them. She anticipated that her parents would hear her diagnosis as "a death sentence" and see her as "sick," as "about to die." This fear made disclosure all the more difficult since, despite her concerns, she saw herself as "healthy" and "living with the virus."

With both of them, I felt that I was going to have to be in a supportive role— and I wasn't ready to do that—to reassure them everything's going to be okay, educate them, be able to talk about the fears that they would express that would be as big or bigger than mine about my future. I didn't feel like they

were the people I could go to for comfort when I'm flipping out. So I wanted
to be in control and say, here's the deal and I'm okay now. And I didn't feel like
I could have done that then. It was just really hard not telling them. It's a lot to
hide.

I told my dad first. On the phone. He's always kind of distant. And so he was
still kind of distant. We talked about it a bit, and he just said, "Well, God will
take care of you." He's, like, born-again. I can't really relate to him. It was just
like, take your vitamins and whatever and I'll pray for you. With my mother it
was more intense. I picked up the phone and called her and said, "I have
something to tell you," and she's like, "What?" I woke her up . . . That didn't
help matters at all. And I said, "I'm HIV positive," and she said, "No, no, that
can't be, you're kidding." She was just in shock. I think she went through a
thing almost as hard as I did. She told me once that she wishes that she could
take it from me—that she had it.

Thus, the parent-child bond can be so intense that not only is sorrow shared
but the pain itself is experienced and assumed. A loving parent may wish to
unburden a child by taking on the suffering, presumably knowing full well
how impossible such an effort would be.

Decisions about the timing of disclosure could also reflect an appreciation
of the cultural factors that molded parental behavior. Howard, the teacher
who learned of his HIV infection at age 44, delayed telling his Catholic parents because he thought they could not be emotionally supportive, given
what he perceived to be a cultural norm. Yet ultimately he needed to reveal
his diagnosis. Silence was no longer tenable.

Now I've told them that I have full-blown AIDS, and so they have to ask a little
more about how you're feeling. And it's not that they're not caring, it's just
how Irish Catholic families tend to be. They don't show their emotions. I know
they care. When I want them, I can call them and they'll come up. But in the
meantime my hospital room will be full of other people who have come first.

But others delayed disclosure because they perceived a parent's psychological limits. William, the married bisexual man, disclosed to his parents
only when, because of his interactions with them, he could no longer hide
the diagnosis.

My father is constantly up on life. He's just one of these happy, happy people.
He calls me up. He knows I can't stand him. And he wants to have these
cheery conversations. After a while I just couldn't stand it any more. And we
decided that we were going to have to tell him. He was a wonderful husband
to my mother, and took care of her through a very long illness, and I just knew

> that this was going to really hurt him, despite the fact that we don't get along. I mean, I know he really loves me, and it was just going to tear him apart. So it was hard. He's the only person I told where I was really scared, I was scared of his reaction. He didn't really react. My father keeps things inside.

An ever widening chasm could thus develop between those who bore the trauma of illness and those who were left unaware. This gulf could be experienced as intolerable.

Those who saw themselves as having been a source of great pain for their parents could also postpone disclosure, yet here, too, in the end meet with unexpected acceptance. Emanuel, who, after years of heroin use, had gone on to earn a professional social work degree, waited seven years to tell his mother.

> I wanted to excel and prove to my mom that her son wasn't just a junkie on the street, that I had capability, talent, and can do something. After I'd done so much, and brought her a graduate degree, and became a professional, and remained clean and sober and acted responsibly with my family, it just wasn't fair. But it was too late.
>
> I just recently disclosed to her. I was real sick when I was younger, and I have strong memories of my mother taking me hand-in-hand to hospitals and of feeling real helpless. When I told her, she tried to assure me that I was healthy now and that they're coming up with new things every day. Then she did something that I really didn't expect: she told me that she had tuberculosis and was taking medication. She was offering me assurance, identifying with me, which really threw me off. For her to connect with me that way, with what I was going through, was unexpected. It was good.

A few found the prospect of telling so daunting that they sought an intermediary to help in breaking the news. When she learned about her infection, Sherri, fearing how her mother might react, waited six months to tell her. Sherri sought her psychotherapist's help in arranging to shed the secret and, in so doing, found the parental support she craved.

> My therapist and my mother's therapist are good friends. And so what I wanted to do was to get all of us together, I wanted to tell my mother in that setting because I was very worried about how she would react. I've known my therapist and my mother's therapist for years. I just trust them. So we had this meeting. We've done this when there've been big issues. I was really scared, I mean, I was just afraid that my mother might collapse or freak out or something, not be able to handle it. I just really didn't want to be another burden. I just told her, plain out basically. I just said, "Well, you know, I tested

myself and I'm positive." And she just came to me and hugged me, and told me that that's what she thought I was going to say. And she said something interesting: she said she was relieved it wasn't something worse. Oh, my God, she said, she was relieved it wasn't something worse! How much worse can something be? Still, I'm glad I told my mother. And have her support.

Yet as we noted earlier, this sense of unalloyed support was shattered when, in desperation, her mother disclosed this information, which had been shared in such confidence, to Sherri's sister.

To disclose to their parents, others called on friends for help. Nancy feared rejection, as she thought she was infected by a drug user with whom she had had an affair. She said, "I don't think I was a bad girl—just a little bit wild," suggesting a degree of lingering guilt. She asked her boyfriend to tell her parents.

> I couldn't do it. My boyfriend told them. It scared me so much to tell them, I couldn't breathe. It's very scary, a very, very scary thing to do. I was afraid they'd reject me, think I was dirty, and have nothing to do with me. In the end they were fairly supportive—very sad, I mean the whole thing is very sad. They've been great.

Such assistance in disclosure was not always explicitly requested. Sergio, the gay man who worked for an international communications corporation in New York, had been the emotional and financial mainstay of his family in Texas. Hospitalized with PCP, he was worried about how his family would confront the prospect of his inability to provide future support and his possible death, and he delayed telling them. Alert to his anguish, his former lover, Juan, simply assumed it had to be done and did it. Sergio reported,

> I've always been sort of the caretaker, the male figure of our family—the husband without sex. I'm probably the only one who left our neighborhood and did anything. And I always feared that if they thought or knew I was HIV positive, that equated death in their eyes, that also meant, oh my gosh, who's going to pay the rent? How are we going to eat? We have babies to feed. And I didn't want to add that piece of it to their whole issue. I was in the hospital and was talking to my ex on the phone explaining that I was very worried about how my mom and sister and all of them would manage. And I was asking him to sort of look after them. And he said, "Well, you know you need to give them an opportunity to have closure. This would be real unfair if you didn't." I said, "Well, I'm not. It's going to be too stressful for me to tell them." End of conversation. Then three or four hours later, he calls me back and says, "You don't have to worry, I've just come from your home and I've sat down

with your mom and your sister and I told them. There were a lot of tears and
a lot of questions, but they are ready to be supportive and be strong for you."

Despite the concern about protection of confidentiality that he shared with
other HIV-infected individuals, Sergio was clearly relieved when Juan assumed the responsibility of notifying the family.

Brothers and sisters could perform that function as well. Patrick, the closeted bisexual police officer, struggled for a while with how to tell those to
whom he was closest, and he could not bring himself to tell his parents. In
tears, he recalled an emotional encounter in which he confided in his sister,
who then took the responsibility on herself.

> My sister told my mother, who went and told my father. My mother was very
> emotional, worked up. At that point she was still strong. She cried a lot, but
> hugged me and I think that helped. My father didn't react to it that way. He
> never confronted me about it. He was a state trooper. He was watching the
> Mets, and she and one of my other sisters went in, and they sat there and told
> him, "He has AIDS, and he's doing good, but this is what he has." He said,
> "Eh, he'll be all right, they'll come up with a cure." I knew that was his way of
> dealing with things. He never talked with me about it.
>
> He had a lot of dementia his last year. He was in the Veterans' Hospital, and
> I was the one really visiting him. I was going about three, four times a week.
> And with all his shouting and yelling, screaming for ice cream and dribbling,
> every now and then he would come into play, like normal. He'd look at me
> and hold my hand and tell me he loved me, "I'm so sorry you have AIDS." He
> knew about it. And he said, "But you'll be all right, kid, you'll be all right." He
> knew about it. He knew I was there visiting. He knew I was there holding him,
> that I was still good, that I loved him and it didn't matter what I had.

Although most of those who had parents ultimately told them, for others,
anxiety and ambivalence led to a succession of excuses for not doing so. One
gay man hoped that the sixth anniversary of his diagnosis would be different.

> I've never told my parents. Last month I went to a seminar about telling your
> parents. I plan on telling my family around my sixth anniversary. I just don't
> want to tell them yet. Every time I did want to tell them, something would
> come up. First my mother's health. Then my father's health. Then my mother's
> health again, with her back. What I'm really afraid of is that I'm going to have
> to be an educator, and I don't have the energy to educate right now. Plus I
> don't want them worrying when there's eight hundred miles between us.
> What can they do for me with eight hundred miles in between us? I love them
> dearly. And they love me, but with all those miles between us, how can they

be of support? My family's like that. You do for yourself. You don't look for shoulders to cry on. We were raised with a real big work ethic, that you took care of yourself, that you worked, and pulled your weight, and didn't really need a support system. Not telling weighs on me all the time, because I love them. I love them with my whole heart and soul. I respect them. I'm thankful and grateful for everything they did.

A few made straightforward, if hard, decisions not to tell parents, because telling would burden parents more than it would relieve the difficulties of keeping a secret. Roger, the former drug user who had told only his wife, did not want to harm his elderly mother.

I ain't told nobody but my wife. Hopefully, maybe, I could get my medical records or my death certificate to be different. I don't know if they'll do it, but it's worth a try. Especially if my mother is still alive. She is 89. She works one day a week. So I want her to keep her condition, especially mentally. I don't want nothing to really set her off. She'd get to moping around and thinking about me dying with AIDS.

In poor communities where use of injectable drugs fuels the spread of HIV, it is not unusual for more than one sibling to be HIV infected. Oren, a 39-year-old gay African American who lived in a shelter, wanted to shield his mother from the fact that he, like his brother, was infected. "The only person that I'm scared to tell is my mother, because I don't know how she would take it if she knows that two of us are dying of HIV. My mother's old. I don't think her heart would take it."

As with those delaying disclosure, the choice of silence could result not only from love and desire to protect but also from fear that parents, because of values or previous admonitions, would be unable to offer support or sympathy. Guadalupe, the secretary, saw her mother and father as cold and unforgiving.

I would never tell my family. Unfortunately, even though they're my parents, they are very backward people that wouldn't understand. I would not tell my mother because I think she would say to me, "You see? I told you to stay away from that man." She would never let me forget. She would drive me nuts. My father? I think he would be disappointed in me: "So what else is new?" So I won't tell him.

The decision to remain silent, for whatever reason, could cause great pain. Individuals might feel bonds of affection but fear being misunderstood, infantilized, or blamed. Jennifer, a 45-year-old white heterosexual who worked as a computer graphics designer, wept as she told of her decision not to inform her parents. For her, given the nature of familial bonds, not to tell was tantamount to lying.

> It's difficult not talking about it, not that I speak to them about a lot of my life. But I'd like to share something major like this. If it were cancer, I would probably tell them. But it's a disease that's not readily understood by older people. I'm pretty close to my mother, and there are times when I really hurt emotionally. I value their judgments, and they're very loving and caring people. I sometimes feel that I'm lying to them by not talking to them about it. I have a very strong Christian faith. So do they. But the judgments from the other side are just something that I don't want to deal with. As a child I was rebellious, and as an adult I was rebellious, and I can only hear, "I told you so." And I don't want to hear it.

Men and women, as they spoke of their decisions about whether, when, and how to disclose their infections to parents, illuminated the Janus-faced quality of intimate secrets. Some told parents before disclosing to anyone else. Others delayed telling or vowed never to do so. Many told because of an emotional imperative, reflecting bonds of love, tapping the most basic of instincts: to be protected by parents, those who had given them life. Yet the secret to be shared carried with it enormous burdens. What, after all, could be a greater source of pain than learning that a fatal infection afflicts one's child? In seeking to spare their parents, those who delayed or refused to disclose demonstrated the ways in which secrets could protect. These individuals also poignantly made clear the role reversal experienced as adult children begin to care for their parents' well-being. But for some, decisions not to tell arose not only from bonds of affection but from feelings that they could not get what they needed from their parents. In such situations, the determination of adult children to keep their infection a secret illuminated gulfs that already existed. The silence simply gave testimony to the emotional distance that characterized the relationship.

Telling In-laws

HIV-positive individuals with uninfected spouses faced vexing questions of whether and how to tell in-laws. Dilemmas arose, too, about who should make those decisions. In some instances, the issues posed little conflict, with both partners agreeing that telling was either appropriate or not. However, that was not always the case.

Since most heterosexual men became infected through a history of injecting-drug use, the decision to remain secretive often reflected a desire to hide a past now viewed with regret or shame. Frank, the former heroin addict who had attended law school, said,

> I have a lot of mixed feelings and fears and regrets about not telling my in-laws. On the one hand, I'd like to tell them all. On the other hand, I'm very nervous about it, and my wife is even more nervous and fearful about it. They didn't even know that I used drugs. We've been together for about eleven, twelve years. We thought it would never be an issue again. And it wasn't. But this is a related issue. How do you explain that you're HIV positive?

Remarkably, like others, Frank was reticent with his family even though he was able to speak publicly and in groups about being infected. In those settings there was regret but no shame.

Others thought disclosure was appropriate but were anxious about the reaction they would encounter. Audrey, the infected Ph.D. candidate, had delayed telling her own parents and let her husband break the news to his parents.

> He went up for a weekend and told them. I thought that my husband's parents would react very strongly and have bad feelings about me initially, like, "you're ruining our son's life, and you're a diseased terrible wicked person." I figured they'd go through that, and then after a while warm up and everything would eventually be okay. But they were very concerned about me, and that was nice. His mom has been really concerned about me, though it's sometimes a pain in the ass, like mother-in-law stuff. Like when we go up to their place, if I take a nap, she's like, "Oh, my God, is she sick?"

Spouses, when disagreeing, typically, although not always, deferred to the preference of the infected individual. Emanuel, who had hard-won achievements, obtaining an M.S.W. after years of heroin use, wanted others to view him as upstanding. In fact, as we have noted, it had taken him seven years to tell his own mother that he was infected. Thus, despite his wife's effort to convince him to tell her parents, he insisted they be kept in the dark.

> I'm afraid that they'll reject me, look at her and stigmatize her, like, you fucked up with this guy. They'll look down on her for it. I want to be able to be viewed by them as somebody who's healthy and doing the right thing. She had an uncle that died from AIDS. And they all embraced him and loved him. None of this stuff that I'm afraid of happened. It's my fear.

Couples typically negotiated either implicitly or explicitly the question of whether or not to tell in-laws, but occasionally disclosure resulted from a unilateral decision. A palpable sense of betrayal could then result. Jim, who had been infected through sex with another man, felt his wife impulsively broke the news of his infection without considering his legitimate concerns.

> Since we lived in the downstairs apartment from her mother, her father, and her two sisters, she immediately ran upstairs and told them. They have been very supportive. But it was very upsetting. Because I felt that it was my news to tell, and my way to tell it, and she violated it. In fact she's told many beyond her immediate family, many of her friends, without saying a word to me about it.

Such disagreements highlighted the discrepant costs and benefits of disclosure, and recalled the dismay Sherri experienced when her mother had turned to others for support, breaking her daughter's confidence. In a couple, the uninfected partner, facing stresses due to the illness and the potential burden of care giving, may seek support from his or her parents or siblings. Yet the infected partner could fear stigma for having become infected and reprobation for posing a risk to the uninfected spouse. Given such competing needs, any simple assumptions about the virtues of truth telling or privacy and secrecy are inadequate.

Telling Siblings

Disclosures to brothers and sisters raised complications as well. Infected individuals often sought much-needed social support from their siblings. Siblings, unlike parents, share generational experiences and might be more familiar with drug use and contemporary sexual mores. Unlike other peers, however, they are kin and can be mired in lifelong histories of sibling rivalries or other complex family dynamics. Moreover, while siblings are related by blood, the norms of duty and responsibility owed to them are less defined than those involving parents. For those we interviewed, the nature of pre-existing family bonds and relationships inevitably shaped these disclosure decisions.

Disclosure could involve little more than yielding to persistent questioning or probes by a concerned or suspicious sibling. "She was just picking at me and picking at me," said Pam, a 36-year-old heterosexual African American who was a drug user. "And she came close to just asking me, and I just couldn't deny it to my sister." Thus, although she would have preferred to remain silent, her sister's insistence and Pam's own sense of her family's legitimate expectations left no alternative.

More typically, individuals chose to reveal their HIV status not in capitulation but in search for support. The decision to disclose to a sibling could result from an unbearable sense of isolation—not uncommon in the earliest days of the epidemic, when social anxiety about AIDS was so pervasive—and a need to tell someone who could be trusted. Wilma, who learned of her infection when her son was diagnosed with AIDS, said,

> I was hustling in the street and just kind of caught out there. And I just kept it to myself—except for one person, my sister. I was afraid, because people are not educated about it and they treat you funny, and I wasn't in a position to deal with that, and she's the only person I opened up to, just so I could have somebody I could talk to. She's my youngest sister but she's the big sister and I'm the baby sister, and I felt really confident. She really gave me more encouragement. I could trust her, we have a trust, I talk to her about everything now.

The decision to tell could be even easier when the sibling, too, was infected. Eddie, a 41-year-old heterosexual Latino currently using crack and injecting drugs, reported, "I told my sister. She died from it last year. The way I told her was the fact that I saw her medication on her dresser, so I said, 'Look.' She said, 'How do you know about this?' I said, 'Because I'm also positive.'"

Commonly, the decision to tell brothers and sisters involved a deliberative process that could extend over months or more and reflected a sense of the obligations to family and the emotional demands one could make on one's kin. These decisions involved complex matters of trust and expectations about openness, questions of how best to retain a modicum of control over the timing of disclosure, and the need to preserve a sense of dignity. Ginger, the former injecting-drug user who planned carefully when to disclose to sexual partners, tried to face these dilemmas by considering how she would have felt if a family member had kept such a secret from her. She had reentered her family members' lives only a few years before, after years of addiction.

> It took me about a year to decide to tell my family. I took the advice of my sponsor in the rooms [at a twelve-step program], and she basically said, "Why worry them with something that you don't need to worry them with right now?" I was scared my family was going to be like, "Oh, how are you? How are you feeling?" and I didn't want that. And then a year later I thought, my God, if one of my family members were sick and didn't tell me—like say someone had cancer—I'd be very angry. Part of this is an automatic thing—the unspoken rules that I have. It's like, look, you're my family. We're to share this information. This is what a family means to me. I'd feel like I couldn't trust them. I'd feel like they don't trust me. It would feel like they didn't feel that I could handle it emotionally, and I would almost take it like a lie, a lie of evasion. Then I thought, okay, how do I want them to find out? Do I want them to find out when I'm healthy and happy and whole and complete and I can say this is the situation? Or when I'm lying with tubes in my nose and turning gray and

they're looking at me in a hospital where I'm at twenty pounds and, "By the way . . . " I didn't want that. That would be a real horror story to me.

I have five sisters. And I had a mother and father at the time. And I just called them up one by one on the phone. I was surprised at the support and encouragement, just total love. There was no, "Oh my God, she touched my children." But I kind of held my breath for a while. They all have husbands. I figured okay, now they're going to go tell their husbands, and their husbands are going to say, "Don't let her near our kids." And absolutely none of it came true.

Of note here, Ginger raised the notions of a "lie of evasion"—a secretiveness that could be understood as a deception—and of "unspoken rules" operating within a family, guiding patterns of disclosure. Such are the complexities of familial interactions that "automatic," unspoken rules—presumably communicated through years of example—operate. As she suggested, the sharing of information could constitute the very meaning and definition of family. Not to tell would be to denigrate another family member and would be seen as a violation of trust, even a moral wrong. The free flow of information was central to the very conception and function of family ties.

Hence, decisions of whether and when to disclose could be dictated by the desire to protect oneself from accusations of concealing one's status. Jane, who was tested when she and her husband wanted to have children, had relied on the love and support of her uninfected husband.

I told my eldest brother first, almost immediately because he has four small children, and my brother was always really homophobic, and I thought there might be some problems with him not wanting me to be around the children, so I wanted him to know right from the start, as soon as I knew, so that if he decided that I should stay away then I would be able to respect that, and he would never turn around and say, "You knew all this time, and you never told us, and I didn't want you to be around the kids." But he and my sister-in-law were both really wonderful about it and didn't have that reaction at all.

For both Ginger and Jane, family rules about candor imposed limits on the legitimacy of keeping secrets. At the same time, negotiating the boundary between the need to hold things private and the need to preserve bonds through openness proved complex.

With siblings as well as with others, infected individuals had to make a judgment about the extent to which those they told could be trusted to maintain the information in confidence. Given expectations that secrets would be shared within families, among siblings, concerns about what could remain private were inevitable. Roxanne, who thought she had been infected either during her years of drug use or through the sex she bartered or sold, felt it was safe to tell her two infected sisters. Yet she knew that, in so doing, three other siblings would soon know. "My family can't hold water, you tell them something they'll tell everybody else." Once a secret was revealed it would flow—like water—without ready bounds. The information could no longer be contained.

However much one's brothers and sisters could be trusted, uncertainty always lingered about whether *their* spouses or intimate partners would preserve confidentiality. William, bisexual and married, had been diagnosed in the late 1980s. He spoke of uncertainties about his sisters-in-law.

> I could lie to a couple of friends but not to my family. It took me a year before I told my older brother, who lives in New York City. He works in the theater district, so he sees this, and I knew he would understand. Last year I told my little brother, who lives in Chicago. So now everybody in the immediate family knows, and that's all that we want to know. And we've explained to them why we want it quiet. I don't think I would have had a problem with my brothers as much as their wives. I know my brothers but I don't really know their wives. I mean, they were very sweet and understanding, but how do I know that I can trust them? To me the most important reason to keep it quiet is because of my wife. If I'm not around, and she's on her own, I don't think it's that easy to be the widow of somebody who died of AIDS.

For others, only time would reveal whether they had been wise to take the risk of disclosing. Sherri, who had reason to fear the consequences of disclosure for her medical career, and who felt that her confidence had been betrayed by her mother, thus noted,

> I was very worried about telling my sisters because of confidentiality. I just didn't trust them. My youngest sister's a writer, and I was afraid. She's been in the past on the selfish writer side. If it's good for her paper, she'll do it. And I was afraid she would write a story about me, and not use my name but it would be obvious. Then a few months after that, she called me up and wanted to know could she just tell two close friends. And I said, "No. I haven't told anybody else. This is my news and you promised. This is my job, this is my life, this is very, very important." She said, "Well I trust these people." "I said, "Once you tell one person, they're going to have to tell somebody." I was blown away because now I had to worry who she's going to tell, who she isn't going to tell. Then she called me up and she said, "Well, I just want you to know that I thought about it, and I'm not going to tell anybody."

Ironically, disclosure was not always a prelude to further discussion. After having told her family and enduring the anxiety over the extent to which they could be trusted, Sherri found HIV too depressing to discuss with them more fully in order to gain their whole support. "It just makes me feel too sad, thinking about it with my family—that I have something that I could die from. I mean, it's just too sad for me to talk about with my family."

Although many found support, concern, and love when they told their brothers and sisters, that was not always the case. Siblings, while not outright rejecting, could be uncivil and unsupportive. As Sam, whose professional life as a respiratory therapist distinguished him from his brother, said,

> My brother's gay as well. He's a kind of redneck, not well-educated person, and his gay life style is extremely different from mine. He doesn't have a lot of gay friends. I don't think he really accepts being gay that much. He likes men. He does his thing with men. But he's not really out. I thought I should tell him. But then I'd go to see him, and get cold feet and put it off, and say, well I'll deal with this the next time I come home. So finally once I went out and just told him, and his reaction was not very positive. It was actually pretty awful. The first thing he said to me was, "Well I hope that I'm the beneficiary of your life insurance policy." And then he went on to describe what would happen, not *if* I became sick but *when* I became sick, and that we have to tell the family something else because they can't handle this. They don't need to know. And so it really hasn't done well for my relationship with him at all, and it was very painful. I was very angry and very hurt. I've actually mellowed in my intense hate for him from the time when he reacted to me that way. In his humble way, that's his way of dealing with it. He probably didn't know what to think or do and those were the first things that popped into his mind.

Finally, some chose not to tell their siblings. Those decisions could come easily, the natural consequence of long-standing features of relationships with brothers and sisters. Larry, the New Zealand emigré, readily accepted his diagnosis and had no difficulty in telling a new partner, but he decided not to tell his brothers, based on the absence of strong bonds of affection. "I don't know whether I'll tell them or not because I don't see them very often, and they've never asked. I suspect I haven't told them because I think I'm sometimes pissed off that they haven't asked, especially as I'm a twin and he's never asked."

Individuals also decided not to tell brothers and sisters in order to keep the diagnosis from their parents. Siblings could not easily be asked to lie or deceive and could not always be trusted to keep a secret. One man described his two sisters as "tattletales," who could not be relied on to protect an elderly mother with heart disease from the news. Neil, the gay man who worked in public relations and was long closeted about being gay, had told few people about being infected. Only after his physician asked, and after seven years, did Neil disclose. He suspected that his sexual orientation was known only by his brother, whom he did not trust. "I've told him things in confidence before and he didn't keep them in confidence. When mother goes, then I'm going to lay it on the line with him."

But however arrived at, the decision not to tell a sibling could be fraught with conflict and lead to sorrow and isolation, as with not telling a parent. Although she shared her family's religious convictions and loved her parents and siblings, Jennifer, the computer graphics designer, did not want to run the risk of disrupting a treasured relationship or burdening family members for whom she cared deeply.

> There's no reason to worry everybody. If I got sick, I would definitely tell them. But I'm not sick. At times I wish I could tell my younger sister. I just love her so dearly and she's shared a lot of pain with me in her life, and I've been there for her, and there's a lot of pain attached to this. She's a very comforting and consoling person. She's probably the nicest person I've ever met, and sweet and kind. She loves God and Jesus, and it really shows through her. Just a touch or word from her is very comforting. And when I'm in a lot of pain I just really wish that I could just call her and tell her, because I know she would make me feel better, just with her firm beliefs and what's left of my own faith, because a lot of times I think that God got pissed off at me, and punished me for being a little too sassy, and sure of myself, and having a little bit too much fun.

Jennifer's choices, like those of others, reflected the ways in which guilt and remorse could necessitate secrecy.

Although infected individuals almost always sought to control the extent and timing of disclosure, other family members often wanted to influence these decisions, molding the exchange of information. Infected individuals then had to decide whether to let others shape and maintain the boundaries of secrecy. Gary, the gay man who communicated with sexual partners by leaving medicine bottles around his apartment, was concerned for his parents and thus allowed his mother and father to advise him about when to disclose to his brother and sister.

> I told my parents first and just asked them to let me know when they would be comfortable for the rest of the family to know. And actually, when I told them I really thought that that time may be never, that they just may never tell anyone about this. I have my life here, and they have their life there, which

they should be able to lead without my influence, I feel. I wanted my parents to have enough time to deal with it. When they were ready, then I knew it was all right to tell everyone else.

However, following family members' advice was not always easy. Parents' wishes should be respected, but if they urged silence, the price could be high. Nevertheless, Ellen, the journalist, for example, accepted her mother's judgments about the relative benefits and burdens of disclosure to others in their family.

My mother was saying, "You know if you tell them, I'm sure you're going to have their support but maybe they might get on your nerves. You're also telling them this thing and it's going to change their life. You don't know if they would want it or not, and it's not like somebody said you have six months. You don't have a problem for another few years and then everybody's been on pins and needles, and depressed and thinking everything was bad. Think about it." And the more I thought about it, that's how I felt. I just feel like it's a lot of sadness to put on someone. I figure, why should they have to know about it? Eventually I thought I'd tell everyone. But in not telling, you're living a lie: somebody could say, "That's not a real life. That's not a real existence if you're living this lie and you're not having a real interaction with them." My brother comes to see me a lot. We see each other three or four times a week. He's very sensitive. He'd always be saying, "I have to go see her because she might not be around forever."

On the other hand, family members could urge further disclosures, and such advice and admonitions could be difficult to accept. Fred, a 31-year-old white man who was married and secretive about his homosexual past, had disclosed to no one other than his wife, his parents, and his physician. He felt that his brothers had little to offer him and he thus chose to remain silent, despite his parents' recommendation. "My parents thought I should tell my three brothers. But I really don't have any desire to tell them. There's no reason for them to know. It's not going to help them. It's not like they can console me, which I really wouldn't want anyway. Maybe on a need-to-know basis when I get ill, but not just yet."

As these narratives starkly reveal, closeness in families may ease revelations or require disclosure of painful truths. Even when motivated by love, those who sought secrecy to protect family members from the news had to pay a price—distance, despite a longing for intimacy. As they sought to integrate HIV into their lives, some found family members gave emotional support and protection that few others could provide. Yet other individuals received little from kin. If lucky, they could fill the void with intimate sexual partners and friends. Those who, for good reasons or not, believed they could get little from family bore the burden of HIV alone. Such isolation afforded protection and security—but of a hollow fortress.

Telling Children

As difficult as it was to tell parents, especially those who were frail and in need of care, and siblings, with whom one had shared the experience of growing up, men and women often found telling their children even more trying. Questions arose of whether children could understand the meaning of a potentially lethal infection in an otherwise healthy-looking parent. Parents, when afflicted by disease, face obvious uncertainties about whether a child is ready to understand the concept of death. Parents also want to protect older offspring from having to confront such a threatening and stigma-fraught illness. As they addressed these burdensome matters, infected individuals generally proceeded to tell adult children, varied in disclosing to adolescents, and delayed telling younger children. Yet this pattern shifted with the circumstances and characteristics of particular relationships.

Not surprisingly, given the uncertainties, parents could disagree about when to tell a child. Drug-free for a year, Ali, who had become suicidal at diagnosis, was restrained by his wife from telling their 10-year-old boy. It was a move he came to see as justified.

> I just can't see a 10-year-old understanding it the way an adult can. I wanted to tell him a few months back, but my wife told me I shouldn't tell him right now. I think we should wait because he has such a love for me right now. He may think I'm going to die. And I don't want him to start getting into that. He's got a young life. He's a gifted child. And he worries about me as it is.

In deciding whether to be truthful, Ali had come to understand the significance of the developmental capacity of a child. He also grasped that, for his son, the prospect of a father's death would represent a profound loss. Hence he sought to conceal the truth.

Connie, a 34-year-old heterosexual Latina, was concerned about how she herself would be affected by telling her son. A crack user, she had once given birth to a crack-affected baby who died six months later. When she spoke to us, she had been drug free for four days because she was seeking to obtain the custody of her child from his foster home. Her need to be strong and to survive long enough to bring her pre-adolescent child to maturity fueled her desire to protect herself.

His father passed from the virus. Now my son's been in foster care for five years. He's about ready to come home. He knows his father died of the virus. I'm not ready to tell him about me. He doesn't really understand too much about the virus. Now if I was to tell him, the first thing might pop in his mind— well, my mother's going to die, too. And he doesn't know how long I could possibly live. I'm not ready to sit down and explain it to him, because all it's going to do is hurt me as I'm talking to him and I'm not ready for it. I'm really not. I just let it be. I just plan on taking care of myself so that I can live those ten, fifteen years or whatever so that he can have more years with me. When I pass, he should be 21, 22, if I do take care of myself. He could be able to understand it then.

But secrecy prevailed not only when children were young. Older offspring—adolescents and young adults—also needed to be shielded. Gladys, the telephone company manager, continued to blame herself because she had failed to recognize that her lover, a former heroin user, was "obviously" sick with AIDS, despite his denials. She had three daughters, aged 27, 20, and 15, and had told none of them. "I don't feel there's a need to tell them right now, because I don't want them worrying at any time. Right now my health is very good. When the time is right, I'll tell them." In fact, when they asked her about HIV, knowing that her lover had died of AIDS, she dissembled. "I said I was fine, and we just left it at that."

Reticence might also result from fears of being rejected or spurned by one's offspring. Karen, the former heroin user now in a methadone program who was infected by her husband, had a shaky relationship with her daughter and believed HIV disclosure might make it worse.

She was raised by my mother, so it's not really a mother, it's like more of a sister thing. She thinks I'm her sister. I feel it's something she'll throw up in my face when she'll get mad. She'd say, "You're AIDS," something like that, or "Hey, you got HIV, don't come around my kids." "No, they can't go to your house." "How dare you talk to me about something, and you got this."

Disclosure could thus undermine a parent's grounds for advising, guiding, or censuring a child's behavior.

Even with children who knew of a parent's life on the streets, explicit disclosure did not always occur. Nevertheless, in the face of silence, they might suspect or know. Roberta, who described herself as "outspoken" in general, had been a drug user and a prostitute. She recalled,

My son was out there. He used to smoke a little reefer. And he used to watch my back when I went and did my thing with the men. He'd stay out there in the hotel with my husband, while I went upstairs and did my thing and came back down. They asked me was I all right. I guess he understood that I needed the money. I was just making the money, buying what I need for the house. My son probably knows that I'm infected, but I wouldn't say anything. But he has a feeling. I know he does. I could tell. You know how you know your kids? He knows. I want to tell him. But then my sister says, "If you tell him you don't know how he would act." When it's the right time, I'll tell him. And I might not tell him.

Parents could thus procrastinate in the hope that their children would not turn on them. Reticence in the face of suspicion allowed parents to maintain their psychological defenses of denial and to minimize the importance of the issue.

Yet disclosure could be unavoidable—the consequence of clear evidence of a parent's impending demise. For José, hospitalized in critical condition, that was the case for his children, aged 10, 12 and 17.

They found out the night I got sick. They had to take me to the hospital. They were told, "Your father's in grave condition. He's going to pass away." They had to send them up to me to say their final farewells, and they asked during that time what's wrong. And they were told that I had complications, crypto-meningitis, because of the HIV virus.

Parents could also disclose because of their own unique needs. Charlene, a drug user, explained why she had told her 22-year-old son.

One time when I had come out of detox, I had wanted to be clean, and he was still using and had no regard for what I was saying. "Don't have people in the house," I told him. "You don't have the virus, but I do and I need to be clean, I need to get away from this." I ended up leaving him because of it. I said, "I don't want to die. I don't want to die like this." But he was negative, and it didn't mean anything to him.

Parents in search of a confidante also could disclose to their children, which then opened the way to a host of emotional encounters. Offspring could react with fear, anger, or denial. Guadalupe, who had been infected by a lover and would never tell her parents, found disclosure to her adult son and school-aged daughter trying.

I had a hard time telling my son. I needed to tell somebody, and I really wanted to tell him. I just didn't know how he was going to react. My son and I are very close, and I felt that my telling him would do something to him; he would probably be afraid to leave home because he didn't want to leave

Mom. And I didn't want to do that to him. I ended up telling him. Unfortunately it was under some very bad circumstances. We had had an argument the day before, and he was packing to move out, and so I felt I just needed to tell him. He got very upset, very angry. He cried. He said he didn't want me to die. He was angry. He asked me why did I wait so long to tell him. And I told him that I didn't think he was ready to know at the time. I told him, but unfortunately not under the right circumstances. In the beginning we really didn't talk about it too much, which I had a problem with. I wanted him to know and to talk to somebody about it, but nobody wanted to talk about it. So I really didn't push it. I left it alone. But I was very angry and said, "You are afraid to talk about it, because if you don't talk about it then Mom is going to be okay, and nothing is going to happen and she's not going to be sick. So we're not going to talk about it. You act as though this is not happening or it doesn't exist."

Given Guadalupe's experience with her son, she was especially concerned about telling her young daughter. Ultimately an intermediary interceded—in this instance, a school counselor who concluded that disclosure was imperative.

My biggest burden was telling my daughter. And unfortunately she suspected for about two or three years, but just never said anything. The brother that I have living at home is a hemophiliac, and now has AIDS, and because I talk and know about it so much, and also because of some of the friends I have, she suspected. It happened through a school counselor she had been talking to for some time. And it was disguised as more concern for my brother, her uncle, whom she loves very much, her favorite uncle, and I think it got to the point where she just had to come out and say to the counselor that she suspects her mom is HIV positive, because she sees the medicines coming and all the doctors appointments, constantly. I have a girlfriend who died of AIDS, and my daughter found out when we went to the memorial service, and the priest said it in church. That was a complete and total shock to her. So I think little by little she just started piecing everything together.

The school counselor called me. My daughter apparently had just opened up to her and was very, very upset, to the point where she was hysterical. On the phone the counselor basically reiterated everything that my daughter said to her regarding AIDS and the medicine, and the counselor then said, "Am I close?" And I said, "Yes, you are." And she says, "You are?" And I said, "Yes, I am, I'm positive." And so the counselor was kind of like, "Oh, my God, would it be a problem if you would come down to the school? Your daughter really needs you right now." So I did. I feel a tremendous burden lifted.

Whether parents justified their decisions to withhold the truth from their children out of love, fear of rejection, recognition of a child's capacity to understand, or desire to protect a child from anxiety and suffering, emotional fallout was unavoidable once disclosure finally occurred. An eventual acknowledgment implied that lies and deception, however loving or benign, had occurred. Sadness and concern, as well as anger, could characterize the response. A former drug user thus had to tell his son "that I had lied to him about going to this program. I was going there for my HIV therapy. But I told him it was for drug treatment. So he took it very hard."

As they confronted the emotional and moral demands of family life, those with HIV had to reconcile their own needs with those to whom they were tied by blood. The infected had to weigh the pain they could cause by either disclosure or secrecy against their need to protect themselves from injurious reactions or the suffering of loneliness. Although these disclosure decisions share some obvious features with those involving sexual partners, they entail choices of a fundamentally different moral nature. Failures to disclose to family members might violate expectations of openness, but they do not evoke cries of sheer betrayal. Secrecy—once uncovered—can cause psychological pain, but this differs greatly from the injury that can follow the failure to disclose to a sexual partner. But despite the differences in secrets, deceptions, and lies within families and between lovers and sexual partners, the accounts in this chapter make clear that the moral language of obligation and duty, and the dilemmas of choosing between the needs of self and others, suffuse the world of family ties. In AIDS, these concerns acquire additional poignancy because they are so entwined with life and death.

4 DISCLOSURE IN OTHER WORLDS

Friends, Co-workers, and Going Public

Infected individuals must make decisions about disclosure not only in family circles but in the broader social worlds we all inhabit. These individuals must determine which friends, acquaintances, neighbors, co-workers, and employers, if any, to tell. Such choices, like decisions about telling family, must be made within a social climate that many see as hostile.

Telling Friends

The bonds of friendship, more than those of family, are created—giving them not only special value but fragility. Chosen because of the companionship, affection, pleasure, fun, and shared opportunities they can provide, friendships take on added significance in a society where extended families have become increasingly marginal. In fact, in our study, infected individuals recounted that they would at times open themselves to friends when unable to confide in those to whom they were tied by blood. But friendships differ widely in longevity, depth, and emotional significance. Consequently, infected men and women had to select which friends to tell, and when. Some with HIV waited months, even years. Others told at the very moment of learning their diagnosis.

In these decisions, HIV-infected individuals had to assess friends' trustworthiness as well as capacity to offer understanding, support, and succor. Fears of rejection always lingered. Some chose the security of sharing in intimate circles. Others opened themselves to wide networks, including mere acquaintances. All these decisions had to be made in relationships where expectations of trust were generally less defined than among kin.

Friends were sometimes told immediately. Audrey, the Ph.D. student in sociology, disclosed her test result to a friend whom she had planned to meet after her diagnostic appointment.

I was supposed to meet her for tea afterward. We're like, okay we'll have tea, I have this appointment, and get it out of the way, la-de-da. And so I called her from the office and said, "Can you come and get me?" I was crying. She just held me a lot, and it was weird because I just remember thinking that she seemed so frail. It was the natural thing for her to know. It wasn't an issue of should I tell her or not tell her. At the time, there was some level of comfort in her knowing immediately and sharing it with me. It certainly has been the case since.

Once diagnosed, Audrey became acutely aware of her friend's frailty, reflecting a heightened sense of the fragility of her own life and of life itself.

A few chose to disclose to all their friends. For gay men who lived in communities ravaged by AIDS, such a decision could seem almost natural. "I've told everyone in my life except for my family," said Craig, the hairdresser and former prostitute who had known he was infected for a decade. "It just came about. It was nothing like, 'Listen I have to tell you something.' It was never that situation. We always talk about our tests and our medical things. Everyone talks about those things nowadays. I hope so. They should." In a culture decimated by HIV, discussions about the virus have become normalized.

But particularly in the initial aftermath of learning they were infected, most planned very carefully whom to tell, weighing concerns about stigmatization against the need to share their secret. Drug free for about a year, and in a treatment program, Ali looked back at the social climate that prevailed five years earlier, when he learned about his infection.

I told my best friend, which was hard. We've been friends over forty years. It was hard for me to tell him, because it was something unacceptable then. People didn't have an understanding of it. If you sat on a toilet bowl, nobody wanted to sit after you. If you ate at a restaurant, they'd throw the spoons out—that kind of mentality in the early '90s.

Although many might readily tell a "best friend," others gauged their acquaintances, looking for particular characteristics. Some chose to tell first those they believed could be especially helpful and trustworthy, based on special features. Ellen, the journalist who thought she had been infected from a blood transfusion, said,

I told a new friend of mine. She's somewhat older, in her forties, and sort of removed from the rest of my friends. She's also someone who's studying to be a counselor. So in a lot of ways I felt like she was a good person to tell. I first just tried to ask her a question without telling her. She had lost her sister about a year ago to ovarian cancer. So I knew that she had gone through this whole thing and I wanted to kind of ask her without it coming out, if she knew anyone who had a serious illness that they could die from. I said, "How did you find out about your sister? Did you want to know? Did you want her to tell you or . . ." And then she's like, "What are you getting at? Why are you asking me this?" Then I kind of told her and she started crying. She was very supportive: "Look I'm going to be there for you and you're going to get through this." I feel like she was saying she felt like there was a reason why she and I became friends.

Although she believed she had made a good choice, Ellen proceeded carefully, probing as she went, acting cautiously on her initial decision.

In selecting whom to tell, many chose someone also diagnosed with HIV. Such individuals were safe to tell, as it was assumed they would not be rejecting. Roxanne, who feared one of her partners would try to kill her, was especially closed to others about her infection, yet trusted another infected woman.

I don't tell people, because I think it's personal. It's nobody's business but my own. Sometimes you tell people things like that, they get funny, uptight. But she said that she's HIV, so I thought about it. I said, now I wonder if I should say a thing about this or not. So then I decided, what the hell. It may even be good for me. Maybe somewhere inside I don't want to tell nobody, but then again I may release something in me by speaking about it.

Fellow HIV-positive individuals could also offer particular comradeship and knowledge, having shared the problems that might arise. Emanuel, who waited years before telling his family about his diagnosis, turned to a long-time friend being treated for HIV.

I have a friend who was coaching me to take the test. He was already taking AZT at that time. He had been pretty well versed and well read and conversant in whatever they knew at that time about AIDS, which was real helpful for me. He was very compassionate, having been there himself. He identified with my experience of getting the result, and he was just a friend. He was like a big brother to me. I lived next door to him when I was a kid. He was like the brother that I never had, and I saw him as a real strength—as a mentor, father figure. I didn't grow up with a father either, so he was all that.

Others used criteria such as shared sobriety in making their selections. Ginger, the former injecting-drug user who felt that "unspoken rules" dictated that she disclose to her family—that the rule of kinship mandated openness—decided with her boyfriend to tell only those friends who had also given up drugs. The ability to accept her diagnosis also became a criterion for the continuation of these friendships. At the same time, she, like many others with HIV infection, sought to protect herself from overbearing concern that, though well meant, could feel suffocating.

> My friends really consisted of people that I was in recovery with, and my thought was if they can't take it, then I don't want them as friends. That's what gave me the courage to go forward. And so one by one on different days, when I could have privacy with a friend, I would tell them. I got total support. One thing that I absolutely didn't want was sympathy.

While many thus carefully planned when to tell friends, others did not. For Jennifer, the computer graphics designer, disclosures often just "came out." "The moment that I'm telling these people, it's feeling right for me to tell them . . . that they're going to be somewhat—if not very—receptive to what I'm saying." She also called a gay friend she had known for twenty-five years. "I knew sooner or later I would tell him, I just wasn't sure when I wanted to, and it just sort of rolled out."

Like telling partners, telling a friend was sometimes necessitated by the desire to preserve a friendship threatened by silence and by strange, otherwise inexplicable behaviors and moods. Jennifer ultimately confided in a friend at work—a setting that can limit the amount of personal information that gets shared.

> This woman couldn't understand why I would break down and cry all the time, and I didn't want her to think that I was just this weepy person. So I told her the reason. And it was a good thing, because the relationship got a lot more solid. She was very inquisitive. She didn't know anything about AIDS. She was coming from zero and wanted to be educated. Because I didn't fit her description of what an AIDS person looks like.

Clearly, in some social networks, where HIV was less common and disclosure more surprising, there were additional obstacles—the need for education. Yet those very obstacles could provide the occasion for reducing irrational fears and perceived threats.

Others told friends because HIV had radically altered their lives and they could not tolerate the dissimulation required to pretend that nothing had changed. With her husband's support and concurrence, Jane, who had been tested when they wanted to have children, decided to tell her friends.

> Our decision was based on the fact that our lives had completely, unalterably, irrevocably changed from the day that we found out. We weren't the same

people anymore. And we didn't want to be leading two lives, one life of, oh, everything's fine, nothing's changed, and one life of this nightmare that had suddenly happened. And we decided we wanted the support of our friends and family, and if they weren't willing to support us we didn't want to maintain the relationship. It was nothing to be ashamed of. Although it took me a while to get beyond that, I was not going to hide it.

Not to tell would have been to have two selves, each with different conversations and feelings.

The death of an infected loved one, which ended the need to protect that person's privacy, could also trigger wider divulgence. Regina told all her friends only after her 7-year-old son had died of AIDS. "Especially after Timothy died, it became a lot easier for me to speak on it. Before, maybe because he was still here and was involved, I felt that it should be private. But now that he's gone, I let friends know. And I don't feel the shame that I somehow felt when he was alive."

With friends as with family, individuals varied in *what* they disclosed—divulging a spectrum of information from full to partial truth. As we have seen, some tried to frame the news about their infection as positively as possible, not only disclosing but providing information about prognosis and the meaning of the HIV test. At times the optimism contrasted starkly with what was widely understood to be the clinical prospects. Ginger tried to strike an optimistic chord when she told others. "Whenever I told them it was always with a, 'Now listen, you have to understand that this doesn't really mean anything, this is just a blood test, I could live happily ever after, for the rest of my life.'"

Others chose obfuscation, with all of its complex potential meanings. A few masked the nature of their malady, to obtain a benefit of disclosure—the sick role—while protecting themselves from the stigma of HIV. William, who as a bisexual married man had long dealt with half truths in his social lives, initially told close friends that he was "sick," but not with AIDS. That decision, in time, created its own burdens.

What we did on the advice of a counselor, because we felt so alone with this, was tell some friends "our little cancer lie"—which I'm very uncomfortable about. It felt good because I could cry in front of my friends. They could hold me. So I got a little instant gratification. But the problem is that I haven't felt like I could tell them the truth since then. I feel like the more time goes by, the deeper the hole I've dug for myself. And my question is, do I just go through this and die, and they don't ever know? Or should I be telling them and try to explain to them why I lied? They probably would understand. But I don't feel it's worth taking the risk of them letting it out accidentally.

Yet the size of the lie haunted him. "It's no problem with little lies. Everybody lies. It's just that my whole persona is just not me, I mean, what I've presented to people. I think that's what bothers me." In distinguishing between "little" and more fundamental lies, he knew that the practical and moral implications of each differed. Big lies could consume one's life. Such lying could entail enormous psychological costs and sustained expenditures of psychic energy in maintaining a false self, and could "eat him up."

Others refused to lie but were willing to withhold the truth from friends. Elise—who would ultimately break the mold of caution by going public—initially, when asked, denied having AIDS, because she was "just" HIV positive but had no AIDS-defining diagnoses.

> In the past, if people asked me if I had AIDS, it was easy for me to say, "No, I don't have AIDS," because I didn't have AIDS. I was feeling fine. I felt I wasn't lying. I'm a lawyer, too, so I know about admission and lying and not lying, and it's very hard for me to sit there and say to somebody, "No, I don't have AIDS," and know that I do have it, because of the consequences of that. Especially with somebody you care for, it's a relationship that you are jeopardizing. That never happened to me. When the CDC changed the definition of AIDS to people with 200 T-cells, and I had had herpes, bronchitis, sinus, and some vaginal kind of candidiasis, I could no longer say I didn't have AIDS. I am now officially a person with AIDS. So I felt I was lying if I said to someone, "No, I don't have AIDS."

For her, the moral, legal, and interpersonal consequences of lying and withholding the truth differed dramatically. Even though withholding, too, involved deceit, lying clearly earned unique moral and legal censure.

But whether infected individuals told broadly or selectively, immediately after learning their diagnosis or over extended periods, they had to contend with reactions to the news. In its least desirable form, concern could take on dimensions suggesting that a still asymptomatic individual was at death's door. William and his wife decided to shed their "cancer lie" with at least one couple, who then expressed concern that felt suffocating and overbearing.

> We just recently tested the waters and, for my wife's sake, told some friends of hers. My wife has felt very alone with this. She just felt that she needed to speak, to have somebody that she could tell the truth to. So we tried these friends. Just this past week we were discussing that we're just not sure wheth-

er it was the right thing. I will say it was nice to be honest. They were genuinely very warm and cried their eyes out and were very sweet to me, and I appreciated that. But I still think everybody, when they hear that, reacts like we did: they think you're going to die tomorrow. I believe we can trust them, but they're trying too hard to help.

People with HIV did not want to be feared or to be seen as failures or without hope. As we have noted in discussing disclosure to families, those who saw themselves as "living with AIDS" or "living with HIV" refused to be forced into the sick role, seen as terminally ill. They implicitly shared the view of many AIDS activists who rejected the status of "victims." Jennifer said,

I told a friend that I was HIV positive. I was embarrassed. She was in a great relationship with a wonderful guy and had a wonderful life ahead of her. And I was embarrassed because I woke up with this drekky guy and was in a situation that I was fighting really hard to get myself out of. And I'd really fucked up my life by getting infected and not using good judgment. But she's very supportive and we're still very good friends. Still, she treats me a little bit differently. She washes her hands a little bit more often. When she says, "How are you?" it's a little more than how *are* you. I think there's pity and I don't want to be pitied. I don't want people saying, "You pathetic soul." People think that it's hopeless and that there is no life. But I do believe that there is life and there is hope.

Thus, even before the development of effective antiretroviral therapies, conflicting views of prognosis shaped the responses of the infected and those in whom they confided.

In contrast, the effort to avoid hovering could also misfire. Audrey, who was well-educated, now a Ph.D. student, had firm ideas about what she needed. She described how a friend had let her down.

She wouldn't talk about it and finally I confronted her on it. She said, "Oh, well, I didn't want to bring it up and remind you." Well, fuck you, like I forgot? Thank you very much. She's really a weird person anyway. She told me a story about when she met somebody whom she was really attracted to. He told her that he was positive. She said to him that she really did care for him. She really liked him, but she couldn't get involved with him because she couldn't do that to herself, because he was going to get sick and die and it would be such a painful thing for her to go through. That really pissed me off. Not only that she made that decision. But to tell him and tell me! Like, am I supposed to comfort you?

Such disappointment—the result of a confidante's own fears, need for denial, and effort at minimization—could leave those with HIV feeling very alone.

The most painful responses from friends took the form of outright rejection. In turning their backs, such friends produced the very condition that the act of disclosure was designed to overcome—isolation. The rejection could even come from someone who had acted in ways that seemed open to people with AIDS. As Aaron, the gay artist, said,

> I had a friend who was a good friend before I found out my status. She was a good friend of my ex-lover and he became sick, and I told her my status once I found out. We saw each other periodically while my ex-lover was sick, before he died, and after I told her. And we live in different cities, so when we saw each other we would spend a few hours talking very intensely, and I always had a good feeling about it. But then I didn't hear from her. We stopped having contact. That surprised me, because it was a fairly solid friendship for many years. It really saddened me. It's a loss, not from someone dying, but a loss of a friendship. I realized she couldn't deal with it so she stopped calling.

In this instance, grief was more likely than cruelty to have occasioned the sudden withdrawal. But while such explanations of rejection might have moral significance, they often mattered little to those who nonetheless found themselves abandoned. Indeed, such justifications could highlight a sense of powerlessness. After all, it was possible to confront and alter one's own defenses in facing difficult situations. But what could one do to change the defenses employed by others?

Such spurning also resulted from scientifically groundless fears of HIV being transmitted to young children. Frank, the former drug user who had attended law school, had, along with his wife, experienced unexpected rejection when disclosing to friends.

> I think that for the most part I've been treated fine and great by people. Most of my friends know all about it. But I have a friend who had a baby recently who was sickly. Since he had the baby he hasn't called. And I'm sure he had people to his house to see the baby, and we weren't invited. I wondered if it's because of my HIV status. Maybe he's afraid I might transmit something to the baby. It's very strange. I get angry, and I'm thinking about calling him up and discussing it.

But he intimated that to confront such rejection could be forbidding.

Ostracism could also occur without obvious explanation or cause. Frank went on to describe the painful response his wife had endured, as a result of which she had had to rethink the virtue of disclosure.

> My wife had a bad experience with telling a friend about it, who rejected her totally as a result—a long-standing friend. They went to social work school together. She was also a therapist, and on top of that had a lot of friends who were gay and had AIDS, and it was shocking really. And the worst part about it was there was no explanation. After my wife told her, this woman just literally never spoke to her again. Refused to call us after that. So we never really understood. My wife had that bad experience and that has deterred her and made her fearful of revealing it to anybody who didn't know already, because she has other friends who she hasn't told.

Although the social climate surrounding AIDS had improved since the epidemic's first years, fears of rejection and discrimination—a legacy of the early period and of lingering hostilities—still compelled many to lie. Jennifer felt she had to pay the price of dissembling about her status to preserve a valued friendship.

> There is a man I've known for twenty-five years. We're very good friends and have remained good friends over the years. We go out to dinner maybe once a week, once every other week. He works in the theater business and we often talk about dancers dying and designers and stuff like that and the AIDS epidemic. And he's just so off base about a lot of his beliefs. There are times when I've had to say, "But you're wrong," and he'll say, "Well, how do you know?" And at one point he said, "Well, you're not HIV positive or anything like that I hope?" And I had to say, "No," because that would have affected the relationship because of the way that I have seen him talk about this, and how strongly he feels that people who contract the disease should have known better—everything my mother would have said to me. My estimation of him over the last couple of years has gone down. For selfish reasons I don't tell him because I think he would reject me. And I do want to preserve what he thinks about me in his own mind. He's got a crush on me, he says he loves me, and right now I can't afford to turn people away.

Strikingly, because of embarrassment, Jennifer believed she had to hold on to a relationship in which she bore the burden of her illness alone.

The choice of silence resulted not only from the circumstances surrounding AIDS but from prior experiences. For example, some gay or bisexual men needed to hide their HIV status as they had previously hidden their homosexuality. Neil, for instance, worked in public relations and had disclosed his HIV status to very few people in the ten years since he was diagnosed. In fact, he had not even told the executor of his will. He offered a host of reasons to remain silent. His unusual secretiveness resulted in part from the homophobia that had defined his early life. "Realizing I was gay when I was 12 and growing up as long ago as I did down South, that was just unspoken. You didn't talk about it, and it's a big part of your life, even though at the time I lied to myself and said, well, you know your sexual feelings are only a very small part of who you are." The need to "keep things close to the vest" also led Neil and others to resist disclosure.

> First of all, telling is letting go, I lose control over who knows. And it's always the wrong occasion. I think maybe I invent reasons why I don't tell people. I don't really have really good reasons, except it just goes back to this thing of devoting so much time of your life to AIDS, and you want it not to encroach too much if you can help it. Just going to the doctor, getting bad results, having to deal with that, having friends die. It's a great emotional burden that I resent.

To tell was seen as almost magically empowering the virus, permitting it to affect and define one's life. Neil continued,

> I think there's some kind of superstition working there. I'm not a superstitious person, but then somewhere I'm thinking if you tell people this, does that mean that you're also telling yourself that you have AIDS? So maybe you're not admitting this to yourself. I guess I wonder how I'm dealing with it if I'm not telling my friends. Am I in denial? Maybe it's very healthy, because I feel healthy. Why should I put myself in a position where I think of myself as a sick person, when I'm not? I mean, a sick person is incapacitated in some way, and I don't right now see myself that way. You have to live a normal life as much as you can, so telling people about the disease means you're letting the virus encroach on your life even more. That's less of a normal life and more of being an invalid, or someone to be pitied or shunned. I don't want to be treated differently.

Others, as we have noted, echoed this theme of eschewing "pity," which in contemporary usage has come to imply showing slight contempt for a person as inferior or immoral.

Stigma arising from other sources also impeded disclosure. For example, Donna, the lesbian and long-time drug user who disclosed to her lover only when they were moving in together, saw HIV as "a big secret"—one that was with her "all the time." She didn't tell, because it would be "extra baggage." "For the longest time it was seen as a gay men's disease. Or if you weren't a gay man, then you were a woman who was getting bumped in the butt, or you were shooting drugs or were a loose woman. There's a whole bunch of stuff and I just don't need the extra baggage. I got enough as it is—being on welfare, being poor."

Whatever the reasons, fears, or rationalizations, some individuals told virtually none of their friends. Andrew, the gay chef, told almost no one in the six years since he had learned he was infected. "I think in total I've told three friends, that's it. I don't talk about it, because people still are ignorant. I've not told any straight people. Forget about it. I just can't get into that."

Health care workers faced particular difficulties, as courts upheld discrimination against them because of the remote possibility that they could inadvertently expose patients to HIV. Sherri worked in a hospital, and consequently would not disclose the truth to any associates, as it might endanger her career. However necessary, her decision created difficulties as well.

> I'm in a women's support group. But other than that, nobody knows—none of my doctor friends. My best friends don't know. It becomes very burdensome, because I feel like I'm walking on eggs a lot. Most of my friends are doctors, and we're out for dinner or something, and I feel like there's this big, enormous thing that I have that is just a big part of my life, and that makes me feel just kind of uncomfortable. I find sometimes when the dinner conversation turns to trivial things, things that are important but not life-and-death issues, I get annoyed. I usually keep my mouth shut.

The onerousness of silence could thus be measured not only in terms of relative isolation but in the ways it diminished the ease of ordinary quotidian exchanges. The enormity of Sherri's secret—bearing on matters of life and death—made the concerns of her colleagues, the stuff of everyday life, intolerably trivial.

Finally, some told no one because they had no one to tell, their social networks having been devastated by AIDS. "They're all gone," said Wilma, the homeless woman who was diagnosed when she gave birth to her son, and who had managed to survive in her Harlem community. "One minute they was okay, the next minute, gone."

With friends as with family members, HIV-positive individuals thus had to struggle with conflicting needs: to protect themselves through silence and to talk about being infected. In choosing whom to tell, they redefined the extent, significance, and meaning of their friendships. Whereas some could tolerate a relationship within which they kept an important secret, others found such encounters false and unbearable. In the face of HIV, some experienced a heightened sense of intimacy with friends, others surrounded themselves with the protective, isolating shield of concealment. Many individuals feared their diagnoses would be seen as indicative of a larger failure, or that sharing the information would make the diagnosis more "real"—giving it not only a medical but a social presence that, they dreaded, could hasten the progression of disease. Those who concealed their HIV bore a double burden: a viral threat to their lives and a loneliness that seemed to offer the only social haven.

Telling at Work

People infected with HIV also wrestled with whether to disclose at work. Given that much of their day was spent with co-workers and colleagues, remaining silent could feel oppressive. But disclosure could result in isolation—and the loss of employment.

Both the personal knowledge of friends who had been fired because of HIV and the general social climate promoted such apprehension. In the earliest years of the epidemic, employment discrimination was clear.[1] Public health officials, concerned about how such discrimination would affect the willingness of individuals to undergo HIV testing, repeatedly cited scientific evidence that people with HIV posed no hazard in the workplace or the classroom.[2] Gradually, the law—first locally, then federally as well—began to protect those with the virus.[3] By the 1990s outright discrimination had become less common, but the legacy remained, profoundly affecting the willingness of men and women to disclose infection to co-workers and employers.[4]

In unusual instances, infected individuals themselves still harbored fears —which public health officials had termed groundless—about transmitting HIV to others. Andrew, the chef, was cautious, wearing socks when visiting the baths. He dreaded endangering customers at the restaurant that he owned and worked in. "I was very careful. I'm a cook, and that made me crazy, because I used to get so scared that I would cut myself and blood would get into food. To me that's very dangerous."

But for the most part, the story was very different. Fears centered on how others could impose additional burdens on those who were infected. Oren, the gay shelter resident whose brother was also infected, worked episodically and recognized the difference between formal legal protections and the realities of the workplace.

> If I'm working and then tell them that I'm HIV positive, first thing: I'd be out of a job. I know they say they ain't supposed to terminate you because you got it. But you never know what's on that other person's mind. That person might

be saying, "Oh, we ain't going to terminate you," but the next week, "Oh, we ain't got nothing to do." That's saying, I'm fired, but they're doing it in a slick way so nobody knows.

Loss of a job threatens individuals not only with loss of income but loss of health insurance as well, with dire consequences for those infected with HIV. Elise, who came to resent the secrecy she had chosen and would ulti-mately broadcast her condition widely, said,

I lived in fear for seven years, really panic stricken about somebody finding out about me, and what repercussions it would have in my life. At that time I had insurance and was afraid of losing it. I was afraid of not finding work if I lost my job. And without work, the opportunities for obtaining health insurance were vanishingly small.

Yet as we have seen with family and friends, silence could impose difficul-ties as well. Guadalupe, the secretary, wanted to disclose to her supervisor to explain the need for time off for medical appointments. But she felt com-pelled to accept a friend's counsel to keep silent.

I've always thought about telling my boss. One of my girlfriends is very much against it. She thinks something could happen in terms of my losing my job, that somehow they will find a way to get rid of me. A lot of times I want to tell my supervisor because so many things happen during work, or I have to leave early or whatever. And so I would like to tell him because I think he would be understanding, but I won't.

As noted above, the formal legal protections for most employees with HIV had changed dramatically since the 1980s, but not for health care workers. Fears that these workers could transmit HIV to patients during invasive procedures haunted considerations of the issue.[5] On occasion, scholars who typically defended the rights of people with HIV urged those who were in-fected and might be called upon to perform invasive procedures to desist from such practices.[6] Courts that had typically supported people with HIV when confronted with employment discrimination were unwilling to inter-cede when health care workers were fired.[7] For some commentators, the is-sue of HIV-infected health care workers was analogous to that posed by the question of whether infected persons had a duty to protect their sexual part-ners by refraining from unprotected intercourse or by disclosure. The most extreme advocates called for the severe punishment of health care workers who failed to disclose their HIV status to patients.[8] Further dramatizing this issue, Kimberly Bergalis, a woman probably infected by her dentist, in her final weeks testified before Congress and in the media that health care providers with HIV infection should be barred from clinical work.[9]

Not surprisingly, a young hospital resident was urged by those he consulted to remain silent lest he imperil his professional position. "I discussed it with a few different people who at the time all gave me the advice: just wait and see where things end up before you go ahead and make any disclosures. And I think that was sound advice, which I followed."

Vulnerability arose not just from threats of discrimination. Sherri, more advanced in her medical career, also feared how patients might place *her* at risk because of her compromised immune system.

> I think every employee feels afraid of somebody finding out, but as a physician, I'm more petrified. I'm an internist and had been doing pulmonary medicine. I'm doing bronchoscopies. I was petrified of tuberculosis. I was literally living in fear that every bronchoscopy I would do, I would get TB. I was working with very high-risk populations in a room that was not equipped. I literally went to sleep praying that the next day nobody would need a bronchoscopy and put my health in danger. I was really, really nervous, and very uncomfortable with that, because I want to be a good doctor, too. I didn't want my medical decisions to be based on something about myself, and that was very difficult. For a year before I left that job I was going on tirades about the lack of proper ventilation. People probably thought I was just a fanatic. But they didn't understand it was a personal issue for me.

Rather than disclose, she and other infected doctors often chose to withdraw from practice.

> Right now I'm just not doing any procedures, because of the legal and ethical implications. I don't want anybody ever to question whether or not I could possibly do anything to hurt somebody else. That's really the main thing. Already I noticed when you renew your privileges there's lots of questions about HIV, like, have you been to the doctor recently? I lie: there's nothing wrong with me. "Is there anything that could prevent you . . . ?" I just say everything's fine.
>
> I'm healthy. But I don't want anybody to ever question my practice. My advice is that nobody should ever let their co-workers know, regardless of what profession. It's private business that I just want to keep private. I think if I was a lawyer or an artist, I'd keep it private too. It is hard not to tell people, but I think the alternative is worse.

Health care professionals were not alone, however, in remaining silent at work after observing stigmatization of others with HIV. Gladys, the telephone company business manager, explained her decision to keep silent at work.

> People don't understand, they really don't. Even though it's almost impossible to isolate a person in the office, I've seen them isolate a guy who just recently died of this disease, and they just don't understand. People are just not knowledgeable, which I wouldn't have been either had not I been positive and had to seek more information about it. So I don't fault them, but I can't give up my privacy.

With co-workers, as with friends, individuals also sought silence not only to prevent isolation but to avoid being treated as different, and to protect their social standing. Claudio, the counselor in a drug-treatment program who had kept the fact of his infection from a number of family members, said, "It's not so much about trusting, I just don't feel comfortable telling them and their response, how they're going to treat me afterward. I don't want to be treated different than any of the other staff members. I just want to feel like I'm normal in their eyes."

But silence could seem desirable not just because of fear of discrimination and stigma; in work settings, as suggested earlier, discretion about medical conditions could be the social norm. Ronald, an infected middle-aged white heterosexual—a former drug user—said,

> On my job, when people have health problems, they try to keep it to themselves. They don't want anybody to know. Whether it's heart disease or kidney failure, there's just some things that you don't want everybody to know about. And definitely, with something like HIV, I wouldn't want everybody to know, because people can be very vicious.

In the social world of work, candor about personal matters can be deemed inappropriate. As a consequence, individuals erect and maintain professional boundaries and identities that ordinarily preclude personal revelations. Unlike the world of family and friends, where shared burdens enhance intimacy, at work such sharing can be viewed as potentially disruptive to efficiency and as "unprofessional." As some of our interviewees recounted, even with co-workers who apparently also had HIV, fear and a sense of respect for others' privacy could keep people from each other. Whatever the status of such formal norms, those who worked together commonly spoke of their "private" lives. Hence silence about HIV could well be experienced as unfair, as a special burden. One woman said,

> There is this one particular gay man whom I also suspect has AIDS, and he has not come out and actually admitted it, but he has said enough to me to make

me understand and believe that, yes, he has AIDS. I know that he's been very sick, and I know that at one point he was in the hospital for a couple of months. I've thought about it, but I don't feel comfortable talking to him about it.

So strong were the apparent social norms concerning personal privacy in the office, and concerning nondisclosure of disease generally and HIV specifically, that neither of the two had been able to divulge to the other.

Given these dangers and difficulties, some sought to test the waters as a way of determining whether it was safe to reveal themselves. By discussing the topic of HIV more generally, they gauged the extent to which they could expect a sympathetic response and identified those who could be trusted. Guadalupe, who was reluctant to tell her supervisor that she was infected, nevertheless hoped to provoke such discussions with co-workers.

I wear this red ribbon all the time, and a lot of people like that I wear it. I do it on purpose. I wear it on any dress to any meeting. A lot of people have asked me, "Well, what does this mean?" And I said, "AIDS awareness," and we sort of get on the subject. I do it to see how people feel, and I have found that there are some really sincere sympathetic people.

Individuals working in generally tolerant social climates and not fearing discrimination still had choices to make about disclosure, though more fine-grained. Working for the consular service of a nation with liberal AIDS policies, Larry, the gay New Zealander, described the decision he faced.

I haven't told everybody at work, but those I've told are usually shocked. It's fair enough: for most, especially heterosexual people, it's not part of their lives. It's always a shock to find out there's a life-threatening disease in store. I'm very comfortable telling people. I think that it's very easy for me to convey to them that I'm not trying to shock or impress them or anything like that. I usually say that I think it's important that people are aware that there are people like me who are well and doing fine and getting on with life, and it really is not a problem to me. But I don't tell them all. Some people there I think probably would be a bit apprehensive about it if they actually did know, and I don't think there's any sense in making it difficult for yourself if you don't have to.

Indeed, discrimination could occur even when least expected—and often in ways that could not easily be proven. Ginger, the former injecting-drug user, was startled that in a health care setting with an apparent commitment to people with HIV, a supervisor could turn on her.

> I've told at work situations before, and sometimes it works real well and sometimes it works real bad. I shared my status with my supervisor. I had been working with her for a couple of months. All of a sudden our relationship totally changed. We were no longer talking. I mean, she called me up a week later and made an appointment with me to do my review. I had been there for six years, and I always done really, really well. I had never any fears about an evaluation or whatever, and this was certainly a job that I was handling really well. My supervisors around the area were like, wow, this is great. And I was given a horrible review. I mean horrible review, and I just looked at her and I said, "You can't be serious, you can't be serious." I had to run out because I just cried for the next four hours. That's how badly it affected me. It hurt me. And I don't 100 percent say the woman wanted me out because I'm HIV. I don't know that, but I just know that this was the chain of events.

But despite the prospects of such painful and injurious responses, others eventually could not endure the continuing burden of silence. White and middle class, Audrey often felt she was an outsider with other HIV-positive women, most of whom were poorer African Americans and Latinas. Of her decision to tell only some at work, she said,

> I didn't tell people at work for a long time, which was really hard, but I was told by my counselors, "Be careful, don't tell." And I have a lot of good friends at work, so it was a really hard thing for me to do. After a few weeks I told two close friends at work, and that was a major relief. Because I was going to work in a fucking daze. Like, listening to people complain that their rent was going up or whatever: I have a tough life, poor me. And I'm like, fuck you, you know? It was hard, I had my own office then, I'd be crying and trying to hide it, and it was really rough. It would have been better for me to have told people earlier on there.

At times, medical needs made disclosure to supervisors unavoidable. Both the law and the values of the employer could ease such a decision. "I'm not afraid of being discriminated against," said Jennifer, "because the company that I work for is very outspoken with regard to this." Thus she could feel free to tell a supervisor, because her illness necessitated special accommodation. "I started to get very tired again, and I wanted to maybe go on flex time. My supervisor, an older woman, wanted to know why, and I told her. It really caught her by surprise. But they go to conferences and are taught how to deal with all sorts of situations that might hit them from people. She was very appropriate in her dealings with it."

Concerns about the ability to carry out one's job responsibilities could also dictate the decision to inform a supervisor. Sergio, who worked for an international communications corporation, said,

> I didn't tell anyone at work in '89. I didn't think I could tell anyone and tell them they had to keep it secret. Although I had a few friends at work, they were not part of my family of choice, so to speak, except for one or two women that I knew. Then I got sick. I guess it was '93. I was in a really, really, really high-stress position and it was taking twelve-hour days, six, seven days a week. I started confiding in a few people at work. I didn't really tell any of my managers until about two weeks before I went in the hospital. They were getting ready to all leave for Europe and I was going to be in charge of the office for a month while they were gone, and I just lay in bed and thought, they've got to know because they can't go without a contingency plan. I called the vice president and a few other people and said, "You guys are leaving on a trip, you're going to be gone a while, you're expecting me to run the ship. You know I can do it. You know I want to do it. There's a piece of the puzzle you don't know. And here's what it is. And it's that I'm HIV positive, and although I am asymptomatic at this point, I'm feeling something odd with my body and I'm concerned that there might be a need for some attention while you're gone." That floored everybody. Lots of tears, lots of sadness, lots of crying, lots of surprise—I guess that I would be willing to say this, and that I was looking at it in a business perspective. They canceled their trip. That was on a Monday. Friday of that week, I ended up in the hospital. I had pneumonia. The doctors were sure I was going to die. They had the lawyers come in and do a will. Mom flew in from Texas. They were ready. So, I guess that's when people at work were told so that they could come and say good-bye if they wanted.

The challenges of dealing with the world of work highlight the especially difficult choices faced by people with HIV. Work environments are unique— consisting of individuals who are not necessarily friends but with whom one spends a significant proportion of one's waking day. As our interviewees reported, co-workers did not routinely share medical information about themselves. But what made AIDS different—and stood it in relief—was that fear played so large a role in decisions about whether to be open or closed. As the social climate surrounding AIDS has changed and as the law has created some protections, those with HIV infection have increasingly been able to confront the question of workplace disclosure based on their own needs to avoid isolation and preserve privacy. In confronting these choices, they have had to encounter co-workers' capacities for both concern as well as cruelty.

Going Public

Silence and secrecy, as we have repeatedly seen, could protect but also make HIV-positive individuals feel imprisoned and claustrophobic, fueling feelings of shame. Inevitably, many people with HIV felt burdened by an oppressive secrecy that they yearned to shatter; they wanted to share their story with the world, to "go public." Such a desire arose from several motives—from the most personal to the most political. The act of "coming out" with AIDS and HIV could be designed to challenge the damaging social attitudes cloaking the epidemic or could stem from past painful experiences of silence. "Going public" varied in context and content, from tentative steps into the public sphere to grand orchestrated gestures—hurling the fact of illness at a hostile world.

Some who wanted to go public believed they had to wait for an opportune moment when their infection could no longer serve to justify penalization by others. Jane, who had been infected sexually years earlier, wanted to wait until finalizing plans for having a child through a surrogate mother. "After we get the baby I would like to become public about it. I won't have my job anymore. I would like to become much more active." When she was thus freed, she vowed to use the occasion to put a human face on AIDS.

> AIDS is not a judgment from God. It's not this big moral issue, it is just a disease, and people who have it shouldn't be treated as if they're bad or dangerous or on the verge of dying. They're just like everybody else, and they can be touched and hugged and shown affection. I'm living with it. When it's brought down to just one person, the disease has a face, and this is my face. I'm really normal looking; there's nothing scary about me.

Others wanted to go public but felt they couldn't. Sherri, very self-protective and concerned that she might become the subject of others' gossip and that a misstep could end her medical career, could not imagine exposing herself to public scrutiny. Nonetheless, she fantasized about what she might do in the future. "You read all these things in magazines about this woman, and that one, and Mary Fisher," a wealthy woman—infected by her husband—who spoke at the Republican National Convention in 1992. "I wouldn't do that, first of all for my own confidentiality. I'd never talk to a reporter. If I decide that I have something to say about HIV, I'm going to write my own story, but I'll write it anonymously."

Some moved beyond the hypothetical, though still relying on the cloak of anonymity when speaking out. Patrick, the bisexual police officer, felt compelled to change the image of AIDS, to make clear that people in New York's outer boroughs had also been affected.

> There was an article in the paper: somebody had spoken up. They showed their face. And I remembered a couple of other stories where people had spoken out on it. And I felt very good reading those articles. They told me I wasn't alone, that people were trying to confront this or live with it, that something was being done about it. It wasn't just being held within. And I guess maybe I wanted to help—like I'm jumping in here. I was reading somebody else's story and feeling I'm so much a part of everything that these people are talking about and I'm not saying a fucking word about it. So I thought, let me get in here and help them out. I just called up *Newsday* and they came to the house. My wife was there. I thought the reporter would be there for half an hour. She was there for seven hours. I didn't want to use my name. I didn't want to use my department, because it's small, and I didn't want it to get narrowed too much down to me. I feel sometimes that talking out on AIDS is important . . . It's like a "don't tell or say anything" disease. Just die with it.
>
> AIDS is not just an artist's disease. Cops have it. Veterans have it. Neighborhood guys have it, not just in Manhattan. You get out in Queens, you hear, "Oh it's a fucking gay disease." Yet guys are dropping dead in the fucking neighborhood, 30 years old, everybody with lung infections. I've never seen so many cases of pneumonia in my life. The article was good because it helped me not to be afraid, even though I am afraid of the whole virus. But at least it helped me. I'm not just laying down with this and keeping this within me. And I'm not just going to die with this. If my time comes, I've done what a lot of people seem to have been doing: speak out. For me it didn't have to be a picture or a name. It just had to be a story.

Yet despite his candor, he could not reveal an essential element of his own story—that his infection resulted from having sex with men.

Some individuals chose to "out" their own HIV infection only in certain contexts. These decisions could make others in those particular settings uncomfortable. Douglas, a 38-year-old white gay man, decided to use the occasion of a school reunion to announce his HIV infection.

> This past fall was my twenty-year high school reunion. They sent out a request for information about what you've been doing for the past twenty years. So I decided to put that I was positive and had AIDS. And everyone was sort of shocked that I wanted to do it. First, I just felt it was important. I figured it would be educational for them to know something like that, and not totally

cover it up. I also figured that people wouldn't probably look at that immediately once they were at the reunion anyway. I thought it was an important issue that people should know, and that way I didn't have to deal with it face to face as much . . . because the book was handed out the night of the reunion. So I assume most people didn't pick it up and read through it. If it came up, it came up. And if it didn't, it didn't. Plus I had no hair at that point, because all or most of my hair had fallen out, from chemo. I got a couple of calls back from the people that were organizing the reunion, and they said, "Uh, we're a little unsure what you want to put into the booklet," and I was like, "What do you mean, you're unsure? You asked for us to write a paragraph; I wrote a paragraph." So there was this whole thing back and forth, this one guy saying that somebody on the committee didn't think it was appropriate. I was like, "Well I'm sorry, just because she doesn't think it's appropriate doesn't mean I don't want it to be known." It did come up and I did talk to people about it. Then I got some letters afterward from people saying that they hadn't realized until they had read the book. Very supportive. So it was nice.

Nevertheless, soon thereafter at a function at his college alma mater, he chose not to divulge his infection. His hair had grown back and the occasion did not afford the same protected context of a biographical brochure in which to disclose.

Going public could take place over an extended period. As such, gay men saw it as analogous to coming out about their sexual orientation. Often individuals disclosed to ever widening circles. Over the six years since his diagnosis, Howard, the Philadelphia teacher, told successive waves of people.

It's similar to the coming out process as a gay man. I started by telling the people who were immediately close to me and people I knew would be very supportive—close friends. I didn't have a lover at the time. It's a six-year process. And it did not include my family. After that, the next wave of people I told were those who were not as significant to my life but who spent a lot of time in my life—friends, acquaintances, some people I worked with. The third level was when I was standing up telling the whole world. I had an experience at one of the quilt displays in Washington. I was a volunteer for a weekend, in '89 I think. Something happened and I just started thinking, why am I still here? Why am I not a panel? Why am I still healthy after two years, after testing? And I dwelled on it for a while, standing there. And what came back to me was I'm a teacher professionally, but I'm also a teacher-type personally. And this was my gift and I needed to use it. I needed to speak on the issue of HIV.

I think it's important for people to know. It's okay testing positive. It's not the end of your world. It's not the end of your life. You can go on and live. When I first tested, they would have told us goodbye, you've got six months—two years max. And here it is six years later. And now I have a two-year full-blown AIDS diagnosis, which several years ago was also considered a long-term survivor. Now it's two years, so what? People need to know that—to look at me and say, this is a person with AIDS who's working, doing well, and looking fairly well. They need to know that the day you test is not the end of it all. It's the beginning of something new. And also every once in a while it's good for me to recall what my journey's been over these six years. I've spoken on TV about it in Philadelphia. I've spoken in front of religious groups, medical groups, gay groups. So I guess at this point I've been telling everybody, and at this point it includes my family. Because now it doesn't matter whether they're supportive or not.

As with others, Howard's motive was to use his personal example to change attitudes about the prognosis of the disease. But in addition, he demonstrated that speaking out could serve not only public educational but personal psychological ends. It permitted him to recall his voyage, his "journey," his progress, and provided the opportunity to reflect on and articulate the narrative arc of his own experience. For a man whose family was not supportive, speaking out was personally empowering, and liberating.

But the ability to speak to large audiences differs dramatically from the kind of intimate talk that a relationship demands. Social and sexual rejections differ. Howard added, "You know, I can stand up in front of a group of people and tell my life story, but to sit down with my lover and discuss something is just different." Similarly, Lance, the middle-aged gay man in recovery from alcohol and drug abuse for six years, underscored the distinguishing dimensions of disclosure to strangers and to intimates. "It's easier to tell a crowd of people than it is to tell someone individually. Don't ask me why. Maybe it's because you're not going to sleep with the crowd."

Others "went public" to confront the shame that secrecy fostered. Frank, who, along with his wife, had been rejected by friends after he disclosed to them, was no longer employed. He devoted himself full time to AIDS-related work.

One reason I do all my public speaking is that I feel the stigma of society. And I feel some shame. And even though intellectually I feel that I'm not to be blamed for this, I still blame myself. In the dark secrets of being alone, sometimes I start blaming myself: well you shouldn't have used drugs, and this is what happens, and you're responsible. And I catch myself and try not to think like that. But it comes up. When you share something with a group of people, it seems lighter.

For some, keeping secrets was anathema. Rather than affording protection, it caused terrible internal "pressure." Searching for a metaphor to convey the need for release, Tony, in his early thirties, spoke of "letting off steam."

> I was talking about it in AA meetings. I had been there for two and a half years, summoning up courage and battling inner obstacles, and I knew a lot of people. And every meeting, I raised my hand, and if called on talked, about it, about how I felt. Some people said to me, "You know, you should be careful about who you tell." I didn't want to keep it a secret. I didn't feel like I could. I felt like it would be better for me to talk. It was a tremendous pressure that I didn't want to take on for myself. I wanted to kind of let off steam and let other people know. Let them kind of give me something. It's just like my family history; my family never talks about anything. I always hated that. And so I've always been one to shout it from the mountain top.

The desire to go public could arise from other painful past experiences of concealment as well, and the desire to be free of secrets in general. For example, Bianca, an infected heterosexual in her mid-thirties—an Asian/Pacific Islander fiercely proud of her ethnic identity—had endured sexual assault as a child and adult. For her, prior imposed silence rendered secrecy impossible.

> I'm an incest survivor. I'm a rape survivor. Now I have HIV. And this is what's behind my not fearing disclosure—I don't believe in secrets. This thing about secrets is that while I was care-taking everybody and being abused on top of it, I couldn't open my mouth: "You have to do what I say, you don't have a voice." So always cramming, cramming, and I got tired of that, and now I just talk, talk, talk. I go out and give speeches, just talk, tell my story. Each time I told my story, not only did I feel better, but it informed other people and cleared up a lot of mysteries, like in families.

By politicizing one's illness and confronting passivity, it was possible, too, to reject the label of "victim." Aaron, the gay artist, said,

> I started to talk more about the politics of being HIV positive, in terms of being open. It's important to be open about an HIV-positive status and come out of the closet with that. It will help people in the future. So I started to make art about it. I didn't often make art that said, I'm HIV positive. But I made art about the pain that I went through, and a lot of it alluded to HIV. I realize now how important it is to learn to live with the virus and not feel victimized by it

or by something coming from outside of myself. Being a victim is an excuse to just let somebody else create or run our lives.

Going public could aid others to confront their own HIV infection but, despite such public and political functions, entailed an inner struggle. Aaron continued,

> I began to be more comfortable being public, but it took a few years. In my life I often felt a victim, even before this, coming from the family I came from. I often didn't feel so empowered or confident. When I was faced with possible death, those feelings of being a victim or not having control over my life came up. And I realized, and I'm still realizing, that I often feel a victim if I give my power over to other people, or let people control situations. And so making the art helped me to see that in myself. It's very autobiographical, obviously.

Finally, others went public to vent rage simultaneously at a virus that threatened life and at a society that treated the infected harshly or with contempt. Audrey, working on her doctorate, told of feeling "really sad, ripped off, cheated." "It sucks," she said, "it's fucking unfair." She then recalled the pleasure of confronting others in the classroom or elsewhere with the fact that she, a white, educated woman, was infected.

> I like the shock value of it. I get this devious feeling like I want to just say, "Fuck you, well guess what." Maybe it's just a way to direct this vague anger I have about the whole thing, at people who are like me, who think they're immune, because I'm such an unlikely person. Once I was in a hospital elevator and it stopped on the floor where they have the clinical trial—it's a totally HIV floor. There's a woman who worked in the hospital. She had a white coat on. About my age. Looked like the same kind of person as me. And she's like, "Oh, so you work on this floor?" "Well no, actually I'm a guinea pig here." And she's like, "Oh." She's trying to be cool about it, and I liked that. That's kind of what I want to do.

Clearly, the exact form of going public—the specific act and audience—varied widely, from speaking to special groups to giving media interviews, and could even become a work of art or an act of ultimate expression. The most dramatic example was that of Elise, the Latina who had for years sought to hide her infection from others. She decided to hold a press conference in New York to make public what she had so carefully concealed.

> I was trying to avoid people finding out about me, so being sick created stress all over the place. I came out mostly due to the stress related to maintaining this secret. I'm an actress. I felt I wanted everybody to know. I don't want it to

trickle here and there. I'm a press person, a public relations person, a communications person. I wanted to have control of the information. I wrote a six-page testimony, and read it in its entirety. I had the city human rights commissioner speak about AIDS and discrimination. I had my daughter speak. I wanted to use it like an education tool. "I'm coming out because I want you to find out about this epidemic." And so the press conference wasn't just me reading my statement about discrimination and fear and all of the experiences I have had . . . I don't have to hide because I have a medical problem, and society has given me another problem that I'm not going to deal with anymore, which is the fear, being afraid of being found.

I did the press conference. I was in the Twilight Zone. It was like when I perform. The whole thing was very organized and was like a theater piece. And I felt exactly how I feel when I'm going to be performing: the fear, the anguish. You don't know what's going to happen, if you're going to make a mistake, if somebody's going to throw eggs at you, if the ceiling's going to fall. I did the whole thing. There were many friends—a hundred people in that room, and a lot of press and cameras. I mean, it was humongous.

Whatever form it took, whether among friends, in a workplace, or in a community, all these instances of going public rejected the need to impose limits on who knew. While each path to going public was different, reflecting varying needs, fears, experiences, and expectations, all shared a common feature: they sought to undermine the social conventions that had stigmatized people with AIDS. Those who went public not only shed their secrets but made it possible for others to consider the possibility of living with HIV, less burdened by the need for silence, deception, or lies.

DANGEROUS ACTS

Infected men and women must make difficult decisions, not only about disclosure but about how to act with sexual partners. For many, the AIDS epidemic has transformed the world of sexual intimacy from a haven into an uncertain and dangerous quagmire. Men and women must weigh their desire for sexual pleasure against the threat that they could acquire a lethal virus or, if already infected, that they could transmit a deadly agent to their partners. As our interviews revealed, in making these determinations individuals had to decide about the relative safety of sexual acts and make moral judgments about what they owed to partners. Those who sought to lead erotic lives under the specter of AIDS had no alternative but to make a choice. Unwarranted concern could lead to needlessly impoverished sexual lives. Mistaken assumptions about risk could result in inadvertent transmission or acquisition of the virus. How did individuals understand the meanings of risk and safety? How did they view and experience these decisions? Did they even perceive their actions as matters of choice or moral significance?

Defining "Safety"

In the years since the epidemic's onset, definitions of safety have shifted dramatically and been clouded by uncertainty. Sergio—who underwent testing hoping to confirm that he, like his partner, was uninfected, so that they might engage in unprotected sex—reflected on the tensions involved. "I was getting a bit concerned, thinking that if the study's wrong, I need to err in the direction of over-safety, whereas before we erred in the other direction." Either way lay potential error with grave consequences. Howard, the Philadelphia teacher and a veteran of gay HIV-prevention efforts, recalled with a touch of irony, "I've done all the safe sex workshops and I know what you can or can't do, although that keeps changing." Similarly, past wisdom could be viewed as almost comically outdated. Tom, the former priest who became a psychiatric social worker, noted,

> I joined an AIDS service organization and got training from them. Those were the days they always used to just say, "Well, if you used to have eight sexual partners in a month, have four sexual partners." The big and great advice we used to give was cut your sexual partners down by half, because remember the odds were just infinitesimal: it was going to be one out of every 8,000 or 20,000.

The understanding of the extent to which women could transmit HIV to their male partners has also changed significantly. These shifts altered perceptions of what was safe. Roxanne, the infected drug user, said about a partner,

> I would tell him to use condoms and he wouldn't. He didn't want to. And then I finally had to tell him I had the virus. It didn't matter to him. There were times when we had unprotected sex. And a lot of that happened, because at this particular time there weren't a lot of men that had gotten the virus from intercourse with women. There just weren't a lot, statistics-wise, and I was under the concept then, because I wanted to believe it, that I probably couldn't transmit it the way a man could transmit it to a woman so easy. And then when I started hearing more about it, I started believing that I could transmit and I didn't want to be responsible for that.

Here, sexual desire, perception of risk, evolving scientific understanding, and popular consensus interacted in complex ways.

At the juncture of danger and sex, a host of scientists and experts sought to clarify elusive issues and conventionally spoke in terms of probabilities. They talked of gradients of risk—differences between penetrative and receptive intercourse, between vaginal and oral sex—based on understandings of the frequency with which HIV could be transmitted during various acts. These issues only became more intricate following the introduction of antiviral therapy, given the capacity to measure viral levels and the speculation on the extent to which the level of measurable infection affects the risk of transmission.

In the face of changing expert recommendations, many individuals sought to negotiate a safe ground between sexual desire and guidelines or "rules" that were perceived as restrictive, even if coming from scientific or gay community leaders. Craig, the former male prostitute, said, "People are going to have sex regardless, no matter what. I mean, according to the rules and regulations everyone should basically be in a body bag screwing each other, and that's no fun. You don't feel it." Given the uncertainty and potential costs of error, individuals had to decide for themselves whether such official "rules and regulations" were reasonable. George, for example, the gay psychologist, acknowledged that he had "drawn the line in a place that I feel comfortable with."

Individuals also defined safety based on the nature of a sexual relationship and judgments about the characteristics and trustworthiness of particular sexual partners. As Tony, the bisexual former cocaine user, suggested about the women he slept with, individuals may feel safe if they trust their partner. "This is the way it seems like people are: once you become a couple, then they consider you safe, even if you've not been tested." Similarly, some gay men who trusted their partners to withdraw before ejaculation engaged in anal intercourse without the use of condoms. Craig remarked,

> I would engage in anal sex if I felt that the person had the potential of becoming or developing into a relationship. To me that is sacred. With the person I just broke up with, I didn't use condoms. We had a mutual awareness and love for each other and caring. We were aware of the pre-cum and all that stuff as well, but, again, I felt that close and comfortable with that person, and he did as well, obviously. We were not completely safe, nothing is 100 percent guaranteed. I would definitely pull out before I ejaculate. The safest unsafe sex possible. To me it was just like the most natural sex, which was without a condom. I would never worry about, oh he's going to come in me, because I trust him.

Yet the notion of the "safest unsafe sex possible" further suggests the high degree of ambiguity involved.

Depending on the degree of intimacy, Tony was also willing to engage in other acts, such as anilingus, which many considered too risky. "How close I feel to the person, the potential of it being a relationship; you wouldn't just go rimming anybody." Conversely, he viewed a casual partner's willingness to take risks as an indication of unacceptable danger.

> There've been situations where I've been engaging with someone and they've wanted me to ejaculate in them. And of course, I don't. I don't even continue going on with it, because I will pick up something from that person. Because that person is basically a wastebasket as far as I'm concerned, and that's not cool. Besides the HIV, anything: gonorrhea, herpes, the list goes on and on. If they're that open to doing that, then they obviously have something or can develop something and that's not a cool place for me to be, so I don't stay.

At the extreme, the possibility of trust could magically banish the very idea of risk. As Christopher, the infected gay actor and former hustler, said, "I just feel like, if you're with a lover, and you two are together, then that's safe sex. What's safe for one person might not be safe for another person. It depends on your state of mind at the time. In a relationship, whatever you do is safe. If it's about love, it's safe. It's with him and he's my lover and we love each other and we're not doing that with anybody else, so we are safe." Danger obviously haunted such definitions.

Irrational conceptions could also lead to perceptions of risk where none existed. Some had difficulty distinguishing between an airborne disease and one that was transmitted through sexual contact. Paul, whose lover, Van, was HIV positive, feared becoming infected. "I was afraid of catching it. I know it's a sexually transmitted disease, but I guess there's different ways it can be transmitted. I mean, if he had TB and he coughed, I would be worried about catching it." He here suggested a connection in his mind between HIV and a potentially airborne disease such as TB. Carl, the masseur, was incredulous at the anxiety of some of his clients. "I've had people who have been on my massage table who brought their own sheets because they thought the person before them had AIDS and that they could get it from sheets. They think you can catch AIDS from the air. Where they get their information from is mostly fear." His observation about others' exaggerated concerns might also have been self-serving, given that he had unprotected anal sex with many of his partners.

"Safe Sex Is Only Relatively Safe": Condoms

"Safer sex," the term commonly used (as opposed to "safe sex") by AIDS researchers, policy makers, and prevention specialists to describe the protective role of condoms, suggests that some degree of risk remains. Of note, the men and women with whom we spoke more typically referred instead to polar dichotomies of "safe" and "unsafe" sex. But despite such binary characterizations, they continued to acknowledge the presence of "gray zones": lingering danger.

Even if used properly, condoms could break. They might be old. The friction of sex could tear them. Experiencing such a failure painfully taught the limits of safety. Otis, the uninfected gay social worker, thus recalled,

> The irony of ironies is I don't trust condoms. A few years ago I was using condoms [from an AIDS service organization] and they broke—on proper use, too. I thought, "Even *their* condoms." I thought they were the most inferior

quality condoms there were, I really did. And they have their name stamped on them. People put faith in that: "Oh *theirs,* they must be good."

Hence, he understood the presence of risk as necessitating disclosure. For Sam, the infected respiratory therapist, moral concerns informed his commitment to safer sex. "I don't want the guilt of feeling it was my fault." He argued,

> I would say that it would probably be a good thing for someone to know what they're getting into, as far as the possibility of a rubber breaking or whatever. I've heard of people who double bag. There's even risk there, so I guess it boils down to: you can never eliminate all the risk. Unfortunately, it's just not a clear-cut kind of thing that you can always have one correct or incorrect answer.

Knowing of the danger of a condom tear, Aaron, the infected gay artist, also often used two condoms when he and his lover had intercourse. "I don't want to take any kind of risk of a condom breaking, knowing that I'm seropositive, and even with my lover, we don't have anal sex any more or very rarely, and it's always with a condom or two condoms."

Others merely accepted the risks associated with such accidents as unavoidable, a part of everyday life. "It happened a couple of times," said Gerry, Carl's uninfected partner. "Knowing that they can break is the risk you take, you sort of go with the flow. If it happens, it happens. What can you do afterward? I don't panic."

And it did occur. George, who had been tested as part of a group of apparently healthy medical professionals in San Francisco, thought he could reconstruct the timing of his infection—which resulted from condom failure.

> I actually got infected through a condom that broke. I had tested negative and I definitely remembered a specific event with a broken condom and having some weird kind of illness afterward. I put it out of my mind. I just thought it was the flu or something, but in retrospect . . . He didn't tell me he was infected. It's always a little bit easier to try to reconstruct these things, but he said some things that I started to think about afterward—in law school, he didn't think he was going to practice law.

It is unclear whether George would have acted differently had he known for certain that his partner was infected. Only in retrospect did he try to interpret his partner's coded communication.

One way of coping with danger was to undergo repeated HIV testing. As a woman who took the test every six months said, "The rubbers, they are not foolproof." Paul used a similar strategy. "I have the test taken every six months, being that I'm negative, and my lover is positive. Even though we practice safe sex, there are still risks involved." Of course, such repeated testing did not prevent infection. It could confirm the effectiveness of one's prevention efforts or reveal the unwelcome news that, despite such efforts, HIV transmission had occurred.

The Question of Oral Sex

The difficulty of choosing how to protect oneself and one's partners became particularly acute and clear in the controversy over oral sex. Uncertainty among researchers, doctors, counselors, and public health officials fueled this debate. Clearly, abstaining from oral sex altogether is the safest course. But is it necessary to forgo the pleasure of fellatio or vaginal-oral contact entirely? At stake was not simply the ambiguity of the data. Oral sex required decisions about whether to make sacrifices to avoid small, perhaps negligible risks.

Some saw the absence of scientific consensus as necessitating caution. David, an uninfected 61-year-old white gay man who was a teachers' union official, did not want to misstep. "If you remember, in the beginning they said oral sex was still safe. They don't say that anymore, and I've heard a couple of stories now." Henry was an uninfected 58-year-old white gay man who had never been in a long-term relationship; for him, the tradeoffs that AIDS had imposed were clear. "I'm very conservative. I realize this is a killer virus. There was a show on TV about heart disease, and someone said that a pork chop isn't worth dying for, and he became a vegetarian. And a blow job isn't worth dying for." Although he had remained uninfected, he nevertheless noted, "I realize I've lost out on a lot."

Heterosexual couples confronted the issue as well. Jane said of her relationship with her uninfected husband, "We've decided kissing and touching are okay and we always use a condom, but we don't have oral sex anymore—that, we decided, was perhaps a little too risky." Clearly, individuals must make judgments as to what is "too" risky. Some found the adjustment to using condoms relatively easy for vaginal or anal intercourse but unacceptable for oral sex. Audrey, the infected Ph.D. candidate, married her uninfected boyfriend after receiving her diagnosis. Of the choices she and her husband had had to make, she said, "It's just no problem with using a condom. That wasn't an issue, but oral sex was for me. I miss it, and he does, too—but not as much as I do, I don't think."

Some have sought to preserve oral-genital contact while avoiding the risk of exposure to HIV. Although he was unwilling to die for oral sex, Henry could temporize, avoiding the head of the penis. "I've done that a number of times, but not the tip. In other words, you could kiss the other part."

Many gay men, however, cited the failure of experts to reach consensus and, in the absence of definitive warnings, assumed that all oral sex was safe enough. Van, whose lover was uninfected, noted, "I don't think the medical community has given us much proof that it's transmitted orally." Given the data, he dismissed precautionary guidelines.

Some saw the act of categorization and the creation of lists of unsafe acts as analogous to the enumeration of sins. A history of the labeling of homosexual acts as immoral, criminal, and evidence of psychiatric disorder made the state's efforts to judge sexual acts, even in the name of public health, difficult to abide. Indeed, many viewed experts' advice with suspicion, as implicitly homophobic. Oliver, the Louisianan who looked to social class to assess trustworthiness and thus to protect himself from HIV, argued,

> I don't believe all of their recommendations, especially since I've talked to one of the doctors who was in there making up the original guidelines. He told me that there were about fifteen doctors and only two or three of them thought that fellatio should be in the bad category. But to be extra safe they put it there, because even two or three doctors thought it should be there. The others thought it was safe, and I know for a fact one of them does it all the time. And so do I. None of my friends have ever used condoms in sucking dick. The Canadian government's taken it off the list. I don't think our government could ever take it off the list because that would be admitting that fellatio is okay, and can you imagine those people in Washington ever admitting that?

In the face of medical uncertainty, even those less suspicious of the government perceived, and welcomed community consensus, that oral sex was not a significant risk. Against the backdrop of continuing medical debate, Howard sought to maintain this source of sexual pleasure when so much else had been judged off limits. "I think pretty much people have on the one hand settled that it's okay to have oral sex without a condom. In Philadelphia, there was a special workshop just on oral sex. They discussed nothing but oral sex for two hours, and there was a panel of four doctors and researchers and they couldn't come to a conclusion." Van added, "I'm sure there are people who would tell you that it is risky, and there are a lot of people who will tell you that it isn't. I'm just going on what I've been doing for the past however many years, and realizing that it does not seem to be a problem for me. I don't know exactly why, but I've been doing that all this time."

Others explicitly compared the perceived risks of oral sex with those they assumed in everyday life. Ben, who had occasionally denied to partners that he had been tested and sometimes disclosed in code or only after a delay, said, "I don't think there's any reasonable risk, no. I mean, no greater risk than walking across the fucking street." Gary, who said he used to be Mr. Safe Sex, concurred; he assumed that virtually all gay men his age were, like himself, infected. "I don't feel you need to use a condom for oral sex. I just assume everyone's positive in the gay community." Though he believed that reinfection with additional viral strains posed risks, he nonetheless had unprotected oral sex.

Even some uninfected men saw the risks as tolerable. Morris had been living with an infected man for a year and chose to engage in oral sex because of its erotic and psychological appeal.

> I felt like the only thing I had in my life was my oral sex. It was something I wasn't going to give up entirely, because that was really the only expression I had, and although condoms can be a part of that as well, they just never really did it for me, and everything I've read told me that there was minimal risk in that activity.

But he drew a distinction between the risks of being the receptive and the insertive partner.

> People go down on me; I don't go down on them. Because being unsure of their status, I couldn't rationalize the activity. There's always a chance that they're not infected. But then they might be as well. However, I guess because it's such a difficult decision to make for me, it wasn't worth the risk if I knew that they were positive.

In their willingness to engage in insertive but not receptive oral sex with men who might be infected, Morris and others distinguished between degrees of danger in which they were willing to engage. Nowhere was this clearer than in judging the hazards of swallowing semen. As Oscar said, "The thing I think is more of a threat is somebody in my ass. But most anything dealing with my mouth does not seem to be a threat, so long as I take it up to the point of ejaculation." He, like others, established limits in how far he would proceed, not swallowing ejaculate. Community consensus provided the necessary imprimatur. "Practically everyone I know feels that oral sex is completely safe, not necessarily to swallow."

But while in the abstract it was possible to draw such distinctions, sexual passion frequently vanquished rational advanced planning. Recognition of the importance of withdrawal before orgasm conflicted with the desire to linger. As Christopher, whose partner was not infected, noted, "We ejaculate in each other's mouths once in a while and sometimes we don't. It's like you can't plan to do something. It just happens."

Even more difficult was the question of pre-ejaculate. Those who believed that permitting a partner to ejaculate in one's mouth was too risky still faced the question of "pre-cum," which could cover the tip of the penis before orgasm. A willingness to engage in oral sex as a receptive partner without the use of condoms required a determination, either implicit or explicit, that pre-ejaculate did not represent a sufficient risk.

Some confronted this potential threat by engaging in "mutual risk taking." An implicitly shared consent made whatever danger existed acceptable. Neil, the Southerner who had been closeted about being gay for many years and who told virtually no one that he was HIV positive, perceived a "gray area" here.

> We're both putting one another at risk; they're being put at risk if they're negative, and I'm being put at risk for a more virulent strain of the virus. But I spent a lot of the past ten years being celibate. I don't think that's a very natural state. So I'm possibly putting someone at risk, but I think there's much less of a risk, because even if you just have pre-cum, maybe there's not that much virus in it.

Given the widely understood low threat posed by pre-ejaculate and the burden of using a condom during oral sex, some saw no alternative but to assume the risk associated with pleasure. As Craig said,

> Pre-cum is basically a small risk. I would never perform or have oral sex performed on me with a condom on, because the lubrication is disgusting. It's like sucking on a tire. Who wants that? I don't think too many people are having oral sex with condoms on, to tell you the honest to God truth. Pre-cum is not a big issue. I guess it can also be said that it is a risk that one is willing to take. It's not like swallowing a whole load. It's minimal as opposed to full ejaculation. It could infect someone, but I'm already infected and I believe that if we must take a risk then it would be with pre-cum as opposed to swallowing a load. I've got more in my blood system than any little pre-cum would ever give me. And I doubt a little taste of pre-cum's gonna throw me into the hospital or drop my T-cells. I think the concentration level, if there is such a thing, would be higher in a fully ejaculated load than in a little pre-cum. It's like a drop as opposed to a tablespoon.

Nevertheless, after oral sex he gargled "to help prevent disease."

Adults, Craig believed, had to make their own judgments about such pleasures and risks. As an infected man, he had decided that a partner's pre-ejaculate was not sufficiently dangerous to deter him. But was he worried about those who took his penis into their mouths?

> If someone's blowing me, I'm really not thinking about that. I'm thinking bas-
> ically and instinctively that I'm not going to come in this person's mouth. Pre-
> cum and all that stuff goes into an individual, and just being adult, you make
> a decision. If you got a dick you know about pre-cum, don't you? The pre-
> cum thing to me is basically in the same category as kissing for instance. Pre-
> cum may be a bit more risky then kissing, okay, but I mean, you either get the
> pre-cum somewhere or you're sucking on a condom and that's no fun. It's low
> risk. Obviously they're into doing what they're doing and they're an adult.

He thought that, competent to make an informed choice, individuals were free to take on the potential dangers of low-risk sex.

Conflicts over the significance of nondisclosure could arise when sexual partners held contrasting views about the acceptability of even small risks. Maurice, the infected teacher, was sure that pre-cum posed no risk and did not disclose his HIV status to a male partner.

> A couple of times I have had such a strange reaction from the person that I
> told that it's made me wonder whether or not it was the thing to tell right
> away. I was away for a month in New Mexico and had sex with a man. I did
> not tell him before we went to bed together that I was HIV positive. But I also
> didn't do anything with him or allow him to do anything with me that was in
> any way compromising. And then when things got more intense between us
> and we started to incline toward things that would be considered marginal, I
> told him that I felt we had to discuss this, and he freaked out, because of what
> I had considered to be very marginally compromising. He was scared out of
> his wits about putting his mouth on my penis—though not to climax or even
> for an extended period of time. But I think he would have even considered
> having kissed with tongues involved to be in some way risky. I mean, he really
> didn't know very much. And considering that he was in the arts, he was re-
> markably ignorant about the whole world of the AIDS epidemic. My doctor
> told me that all the research has shown that unless the person has tears in
> their mouth that it is not likely that the virus would survive in the gastric
> juices, and that it is not an unsafe activity. My doctor considered it not full and
> completely safe, but definitely a marginal thing. And what I had done with
> this partner was a minute or something of mutual sucking. That was no big
> deal. I was not pumping away or doing anything that was likely to expose

him. I was fully aware of what I was doing at the time and thought, should I not do this? And then I said to myself, I just don't think that this is unsafe. We'd only had a couple of dates, and I didn't see how anybody could not know enough about the AIDS situation to not have thought about it for himself as to whether or not this was something he was willing to risk without having previously discussed it with the person. Since we hadn't discussed it, I figured he knew what he would consider unsafe.

For Maurice, this partner's outrage had little justification. It was a response born of sheer ignorance.

In sum, the absence of scientific clarity led many to accept the risks of oral sex for themselves and dismiss the possibility that they posed a hazard to their partners. In the end, many who perceived but accepted the potential danger subscribed to Craig's perspective, "You take risks because you're human and you need that." But others continued to grapple with larger questions about the extent of partners' moral responsibility toward each other and about whether, in the face of uncertainty or even small risks, partners had a duty to disclose to ensure truly informed consent.

The Question of Kissing

As with oral sex, the question of kissing revealed critical fault lines in perceptions of HIV transmission and the acceptability of very low levels of risk. There was virtually no evidence that transmission of HIV could occur during kissing. Yet because saliva contains small amounts of virus and mouth sores can bleed, some thought passionate kissing should be avoided.

A few acknowledged they would be disturbed to kiss a partner who later disclosed that he or she was infected, and they were willing to forgo kissing altogether, if need be. Tom, who was HIV negative and relied on his partner's candor, said, "Deep kissing in the mouth: I think it would be difficult to do that and then afterward find out that the other person was HIV positive." In fact, he never deep-kissed his infected lover, who eventually died of AIDS.

Martin and I never even kissed. Because when we first met, he didn't know his HIV status and he was protecting me probably as much as I was protecting him. In our whole relationship, we had a wonderful sex life, but we never had oral sex direct. We did have intercourse. I used a double condom in intercourse with him. Otherwise, though, it was basically mutual masturbation. It's not so much *what* you do, it's the way of being. I think of ourselves as having a very good sexual life, and yet I couldn't even have intercourse with him that much, because for the last couple of years he started having a lot of diarrhea. He was just a little bit sore, so even that wasn't there. But somehow, just through masturbation and being close and physical, I just think of it as a very sexual time, with everything else.

The deaths of friends and lovers, and his experience as an AIDS volunteer, further compelled Tom to exercise caution.

I worked for an AIDS service organization for ten years, so I'm probably a little hyper, and I've been working in a hospital for nine of the last ten years. I've lost at least a dozen friends. I have ten friends now who are HIV positive or have AIDS. I've lost two lovers and work as a volunteer. It's stupid, I'm sure. I'm vigilant, but I'm saying, why risk at all? And when someone says to me, "I can't live without kissing," I'm not going to say much to him, just, "I find it problematic to do a lot of deep kissing in these anonymous situations," and leave it at that.

Despite his own stance, he recognized that others could assess the tolerability of risk differently.

Those who thought kissing was virtually risk free were startled by the vehemence of partners who thought otherwise. Andrew, who had expressed great fears that he could put his restaurant patrons at risk during food preparation—fears that few experts would view as reasonable—was surprised during a date.

I only met him once, and he brought me a gift, a tie. And we went out, and at the bar, in some way I kissed him or he kissed me. It was not a threatening kiss or anything—it was just a kiss. But a deep kiss. A real kiss. And we went out and after dinner we were walking in the Village, and I told him I was HIV positive, and he flipped out. And then I realized, why did I say that? There was no reason, there's no commitment, I'm not getting involved with this person. And he got so upset that he told his brother, who is also gay, and his brother knows somebody who has AIDS, and they went crazy: how dare I kiss him knowing that I had it!

In a couple in which only one member was infected, the partner seeking to avoid HIV might impose "irrational" limits. Jim, the married computer programmer who had had homosexual relations in the past, had known about his HIV infection for five years. He was unable to change his wife's reluctance to kiss, although she acknowledged intellectually that kissing posed little danger.

She can say that she doesn't believe there's a risk from kissing, but she always tends to discourage it—deep kissing, I should say. Kissing lip to lip is fine. But anything further than that she will tend to turn her head or find some other way to discourage. During the act, I'll say nothing, and just go along with it. And the several times I've brought it up since, she'll simply deny that there's any problem.

A desire to preserve harmony could thus necessitate acquiescence to unreasonable fears, even when yielding felt painful.

But such extreme apprehension was relatively uncommon. Many would avoid kissing if partners had obvious cold sores, but most said they ordinarily did not "really worry that much." Given the important psychological meanings of kissing, most individuals minimized a risk that was almost too small to measure. Otis, the social worker, remarked,

> I made some decisions, and I came to some decisions by people I respected and who knew more about AIDS than I, from whatever medical point of view was available at the time. But ultimately everything came down to a decision, and after maybe not having kissed a man for x amount of time, six months, a year, because of saliva—no one knew about saliva yet, there was that possibility—I finally, ultimately, decided, fuck it, if I can't kiss somebody, then, not that I want to die, but I can't keep on living without being able to tongue-kiss a man. But that was a decision, and maybe I'm desperately wrong on this. Maybe I'm a fatalist, and maybe I'm going to contract something. Maybe it's suicidal if I kiss somebody. So those little decisions are monumental. So sure he's positive and I kissed him. I was in relationships with two friends, both of them are dead, and I didn't care [that they were positive]. One was sick at the time, and we got into a relationship and I wasn't afraid to kiss him. It sounds almost bizarre on one level, but I said, "Fuck it, it doesn't matter on that level." I don't go around telling everybody that I kiss people with AIDS, but this was someone I was really close with.

The range of attitudes about kissing reveals most forcefully how fears of a lethal infection can profoundly shape choices about physical intimacy, even when the risks are vanishingly small.

Sexual Strategies

In the context of the AIDS epidemic, men and women faced the potential dangers of sexual activities—both those beyond dispute (e.g., anal intercourse without a condom) and those shrouded by uncertainty (e.g., oral sex)—and had to make a series of critical decisions about taking or imposing risks. How did the magnitude of risk affect those decisions? How did disclosure alter the moral issues involved when individuals engaged in acts that were of clear or uncertain danger? As they struggled with these issues, both infected and uninfected individuals chose from five strategies: first, disclosing HIV status and practicing safer sex; second, abstaining from sex altogether or from certain sexual acts; third, not disclosing their HIV status but adhering to safer sex guidelines; fourth, disclosing their HIV status to partners and then engaging in unprotected sex; fifth, and most morally problematic, not disclosing their infection and engaging in unsafe sex. Typically, determinations about how to act were not once-and-for-all decisions but shifted over time in the light of changing understandings of the epidemic, different partners, and varying contexts.

The strategy of disclosing and practicing safer sex was adopted by many men and women. The rationale was straightforward: to be fully honest and protect one's partner as much as possible while maintaining a gratifying sexual relationship. The moral and psychological dimensions of this strategy have been discussed in Chapter 2. Yet for a variety of reasons, not all could or wanted to embrace such an approach. In the remainder of this chapter we discuss the other four sexual strategies.

Shades of Abstinence: Seeking Safety in Limits

As the discussions of oral sex and kissing indicate, the threat of either transmitting or acquiring HIV infection in a relationship could lead to abstinence from certain practices altogether. Other individuals went further and, at least for a time, gave up all sex, even with loving and intimate partners.

For those who were uninfected, the fear of exposure could utterly eliminate erotic pleasure. Henry, the gay man who had said "a blow job is not worth dying for," spoke of his anxiety, saying, "I'm never really relaxed in a sexual situation." Similarly, Oliver, the Louisianan, said, though with a touch of irony, "I've had enough sex so that if I never had any more, at my age it doesn't really matter that much. I'm ready to quit sex, until they straighten up the AIDS bit."

Depression and anxiety related to HIV could stymie the desire for physical intimacy. Ernest, the screenwriter, was still beset with the emotional burdens of having learned less than a year ago that he was infected.

> It has more to do with my state of mind right now. My worries about HIV so dominate my life, or a big part of my life, that it's as though I'm in finals week and I can't think of sex. It's like there's just this big thing there that's taking up that space, as opposed to, gosh, I'm still worried about infecting her, or using a condom. I can't get used to doing that, I don't like doing that. So that's probably a small part of it, but it more just feels like times when I've been depressed or worried about something, sex just hasn't been a concern of mine.

The prospect of death could shadow sexual relations, making them all but impossible. Audrey said of her uninfected boyfriend, later her husband, "We didn't have sex for a while, mostly because I was too freaked out, and not just at the idea of infecting him, but it just brings up all kinds of feeling. It's hard to feel sexy when you're thinking about dying, and this is what killed me."

For some who were infected, abstinence could seem the only morally acceptable path. Doubts about experts' recommendations on safety could lead to the conclusion that nothing was danger free. José, the former drug user, protected his wife through abstinence. "I don't believe in that word—safe sex—there's no such thing. Nothing's safe. Is it 100 percent? No. So then it's not safe." Based on the same thinking, Oren, the gay shelter resident, believed that, sexually, he represented an unacceptable threat to others' well-being: "I wasn't ready to have sex with anyone, because I didn't want to spread it."

Some abstained because they anticipated feeling guilty if transmission inadvertently occurred. Guadalupe, the secretary infected by a man she believed did not know he had HIV, said, "That's one of the reasons why I refuse to be sexually involved with anyone. I don't think I could live with myself if I knew that I had infected someone."

Within relationships where only one individual had HIV, either partner, fearing transmission, could impose abstinence regardless of his or her lover's desires. Ronald had used drugs extensively, but he nonetheless maintained an uncompromising sense of duty to his wife.

> It's hard for me to have sex now. I don't know if I just use that as an excuse or what, but I don't want to infect her if she's not infected, and a lot of things go through my mind: that the condom might slip off or puncture, and then I always think about my kids, how they might feel knowing that I'm positive and I was still continuing to have sex and might infect her. So that plays a large part in me not even wanting to have sex with her. When she approaches me I feel very uncomfortable, and she's learned to deal with that. She doesn't approach me like that anymore. Sometimes I don't even hug her as much as I used to, because I'm afraid that it's going to give her the wrong impression that we're going to have sex. I don't want to hurt her anymore than I have already and continue to do by not having sex with her, but I can't seem to impress her with the fact that it's not going to be like it was at one time. We're never going to have that.

In some instances, the desire to protect a loved one could be powerful enough to produce ambivalence about the relationship itself. Emanuel, who had become a social worker, sought to protect his wife—reflecting his guilt over his prior heroin and cocaine use.

> There was this strong feeling that I had about ending the relationship, a lot of ambivalence, because I didn't want to be the one to infect her, to say, man, I killed her. And really since then, there's been this lingering ambivalence about the relationship. On the one hand, I love her and don't want to be apart from her. On the other hand, I say to myself it would be a good thing, because I care so much about her that I wouldn't want to continue to expose her to the virus and then learn that she might get infected.

But both partners in a relationship could also mutually agree to forego sex. José, the former drug user who believed "there's no such thing as 'safe,'" said,

> We've gotten to the point where we joke about it. I say to her I want to have a relationship, I want to have sex. She says not without the proper protection. And I always tell her I'm going to buy it tomorrow. This is our little joke. I'm going to get it tomorrow, you know. Tomorrow never comes. And that's the way we deal with it. We're happy with each other. I'm more concerned that if I do anything even with protection, especially when she's been negative all this time, the next time, if she was to come up positive, then I would put the blame on me, which I don't want. We're closer now than we were before we found out I had it. We'll talk out little problems. Before, we might have argued. We used to yell and scream and fight. We have a very good relationship now. It only added to our relationship. And now that I'm in this situation, that's all I need is to expose her. It's bad enough I did this to myself. Am I going to do it to her, too?

Here, humor protected a relationship that sexual deprivation might have otherwise damaged. Roberta, the "outspoken" former drug user and prostitute, also used humor when reflecting on the problem. "I haven't had sex in so long, I wouldn't even know what a penis looks like."

Finally, others rejected celibacy, but severely reduced the frequency of sexual activity, because of their own or their partner's choice. Neil, the closeted gay Southerner, HIV infected for ten years, remained celibate for stretches of time. He noted, "Ever since the thing became a problem in '83, I've been very reticent about it. It didn't stop me, but it made me so fearful that a lot of times I'd walk away from a situation." Jim's wife insisted on a change in sexual activity, despite his desires. A Catholic, he had sought and received permission of his parish priest to use condoms to prevent HIV transmission.

Our sex life went through quite a bit of a roller coaster. After about a year and a half she began to become very fearful of becoming infected either through kissing or the rubber breaking—something along those lines. And that went on for maybe a year. Sex became less frequent—maybe once in three months. And at those times she would not want to kiss. She began to assume female superior position and not give me any other positions at all.

Those who found abstinence or less frequent sexual activity too difficult to endure often gave up particular sexual practices that seemed too risky. Ramon, the married former drug user, struggled to have "sex like normal people" as much as possible.

After I found out I was infected, sex stopped. I didn't want to touch her. I just felt as if this was the end of my sex life. Because sex to me is all a part of living. I enjoy making love, and I find it hard now, even today, to have a normal sexual relationship, because I'm a freelancer when I make love, like going to bed, do whatever you want to do, that kind of attitude when I have sex. Now it's, like, straight up and down. I can't do the things I like to do when I do make love, so it sets up a limitation for me.

As we have noted, some specifically abandoned oral sex. Others, including Otis, the Catholic social worker, gave up anal sex because they could not trust condoms. Above all else, Otis wanted to avoid becoming infected.

I don't know if I've trained myself or what, but I don't have that need for anybody to fuck me. I sort of weeded that out of my desires—whatever desires I've ever had of it. It's not worth it, it's just not, condoms or not. I really truly in my heart believe condoms certainly can work, maybe you can use them ten times in a row and they'll be fine, but there's that chance they're going to break, and that someone's semen is going to come up your ass. I don't know if one time will break down your immune system and you'll have AIDS. I don't know if anybody really knows. Some people are more susceptible to a lot of things, and maybe they have more predisposition to certain things, but still it's not worth the risk.

Clearly, abstinence was never easy to negotiate or endure, but fears, guilt, psychological discomfort, or a partner's resistance often prevailed to limit sexual behavior in a relationship once disclosure had occurred. Still, given the deprivation such abstinence could impose, many infected individuals sought other strategies for dealing with these dilemmas of balancing desire and disclosure.

Safer Sex without Disclosure

Whereas men and women in ongoing relationships often diminished their sexual activity or adopted safer sexual practices following disclosure, those who were dating or involved in less committed relationships faced different decisions. Many "don't tell, but practice safe sex."

Claudio, the former drug user, now drug counselor, typified this approach, rooted in the need to protect both himself and his partners.

> I didn't tell her right away, "Well I'm positive so we got to use a condom." It was, "I'm using a condom because in case, because I haven't tested and to be protective, to protect myself and protect you." I did tell one partner, it was early on, and it gave me some kind of schooling, because I was new at this and didn't know what I should tell or not tell them. Prior to me telling her, we were very close. We had become pretty intimate, and after I told her, she disengaged. So I said, okay, now I got to be careful about how I approach that. And that's the way it's been. Not that I haven't disclosed. But if it hasn't come up, I don't volunteer it. But the safer sex has been in practice. I'm being safer, and for the moment I feel they don't need to know. I have the experience of rejection. I don't want to be rejected, go through that experience.

The sting of rejection prompted him to develop his own strategy that he felt still protected his partners.

Yet in the absence of HIV disclosure, it could be difficult to justify the use of condoms. Darryl, with a long history of imprisonment on drug-related charges, had started to use condoms, albeit inconsistently, before his recent diagnosis of HIV, because he knew he was at risk from drug use. Once discovering his infection, he was especially concerned about not transmitting HIV and about protecting himself from what he believed to be the possibility of reinfection, a risk that scientists had not yet demonstrated.

> With everyone that I was sexually active with from the time I started using condoms, the issue has come up, and I would say, you know, it's part of learning to love myself a little, just like when I get into a car, loving myself is using a seatbelt, loving myself is using a condom. I'm in recovery, and that's one of the things that the twelve steps uses: learning to love ourselves. I found out that just the little things that I do show that I care about myself, and in turn show that I care about somebody else.

Many white gay men in particular believed that condoms obviated the need for disclosure. That was true even for those who had had condoms break. Although he had become infected as a result of condom failure,

George, the psychologist, said about his anonymous partners to whom he did not disclose, "My feeling about it was always that as long as I felt I was being safe, and I didn't feel I really knew them, then I felt okay." It was the attempt to protect, even if not successful, that mattered.

In the absence of discussion, many gay men assumed the presence of HIV in potential partners. In fact, when disclosure did not occur, many adopted a ritual of using condoms. Christopher, the gay actor and former hustler, described how a sex partner took the initiative for safety without HIV being discussed. "I was having sex with a man and I was going to go for it and fuck him. And it was, 'Hey stop, we have to use a condom.' I always admired that. Yeah, that's good. Not without a rubber. I think that's good."

The decision to practice safer sex without HIV disclosure could result from nonverbal communication as well. Otis, the uninfected social worker, noted about such interactions,

> If you can't make some kind of assessment that that person is somehow mature, reasonable, intelligent, then it's your responsibility. Maybe you shouldn't do something with that person. If you actively talk about it, maybe that would take your whole feeling of horniness down. Maybe you're in situations where you don't want to engage in conversations on AIDS. But if you can't get the signal that we'll have safe sex, "I know that you know that I know that you know . . . ," then you have to make that decision for that person. It can be all nonverbal. If I got all those positive signals, I mean good signals, and then we go back to his place or my place and he says, "I want to fuck you without a condom," you know, wait a second, you gave me the signals.

Roger, the former drug user, put it bluntly, "It wasn't no words passed or nothing. We went to do our little thing, I pulled out the rubber and I put it on, so that was about it."

The use of condoms in lieu of disclosure could result, too, from uncertainty about the possibility of knowing the truth of a partner's HIV status. "Either it's true or it's not true," said Henry, "but I'm not going to put my life at risk, because it's not a matter of believing or not believing. There's no way to verify what a person says, and even if they had a certificate showing a week ago that they were tested, something could have happened during that week." Others assumed they could be lied to and hence took precautions. Paul—who was not infected although his lover, Van, was—practiced safer sex, taking for granted that partners might try to deceive him. "He could have been positive and didn't know it, or was afraid to share that with me. Not that I look at everybody saying, if they say they're negative, they're positive. But in the homosexual lifestyle, you have to, because a lot of people cannot take rejection, so they're going to lie. So you have to protect yourself."

Finally, some asserted that the use of condoms—a shared responsibility of partners—carried the same moral weight as disclosure. Nancy, who had been infected by a drug-using former lover, accepted condoms as a moral alternative to disclosure. "I think they don't have an obligation to tell you. But they do have an obligation to wear a condom. I think the woman should have some condoms on her, too. It's not all a man's responsibility."

In the end, the strategy of safer sex without disclosure often seemed appropriate, given understandings of the limits of trust, the recognition that disclosure could be difficult in sexual encounters, the belief that condoms alone could afford the ultimate form of self-protection, and the view that partners had a certain degree of moral responsibility to each other. On the other hand, others saw such a strategy as providing inadequate protection against transmission. Most important, condoms could rupture.

Unsafe Sex after Disclosure

Other infected women and men, after explicitly disclosing their infection to their partners, nonetheless engaged in unprotected sex. Frequently, such risk taking reflected a judgment that the potential danger mattered far less than the desire to have sex without condoms. Alternatively, unsafe sex might occur only as "lapses"—demonstrating the power of underlying desires.

However much they knew about a partner's HIV infection, denial allowed people to act in potentially hazardous ways. When Janet—who, like Dolores, described herself as "the black sheep of the family" because she had used drugs and been a prostitute for many years—learned from her husband that he was positive, she "didn't want to believe it."

> The mother of his two children died of AIDS-related cancer, and he was saying, "Well I might have it," or something like that, but I wasn't listening. And then when I got my test results, which were negative, I would say, "Why don't you take the test?" he'd say, "No, 'cause you got your papers." And I assumed—that was very stupid on my part—because we were having sex, that he wouldn't have it either. Then he comes down with it. We were not using condoms. Now we do. Because now I can actually see that he has it. Sometimes his jaw be sunk in, or he'll have diarrhea really bad. That's when it really hit me, because even this year we had sex with no condoms, and I knew he had the virus. Twice we did, but I just don't want to believe it. I guess you'd say I was in denial. One time the condom broke, and I said, "Did that break,

Jimmy?" He said, "No, no, it didn't break." But I knew I should have said stop then. That was one of the times we went on and had sex without it on—you might as well say without no condom. But I knew it. I just kept on anyway. Then the other time, about a month later, we just didn't do it with anything. I guess we both wanted sex and we did it, but it was stupid on my part. But I had the test twice more after that. When those came out negative I said, "No more," I will carry a female condom with me now. I just can't take that chance.

Luckily, she remained uninfected. The denial facilitated by asymptomatic HIV infection could be shattered by symptoms of full-blown AIDS—but, as we have just seen, that was not always the case.

Uninfected individuals could also feel that they must be "resistant" to the virus if they hadn't yet become infected—suggesting yet another form of denial. Karen, for example, who was eventually infected by her partner, at first thought she must be "immune" to his virus.

My boyfriend was diagnosed in '85, but I really wasn't too familiar with it and we were still having unprotected sex. When I started in the research study in '88 or '89, they started taking the blood, and it came back negative the first two times. And then the next six months it started coming back inconclusive. Then I knew that I was infected. We continued to have unprotected sex. I don't know why I thought this way, but I thought maybe because I was negative then, maybe I was doing something right. I said, "Well, I'm going to be with this man I think for the rest of my life, so maybe I don't have to, because I should have been infected a long time ago." The condom didn't feel right, he couldn't do it or it caught us at a moment of just hot passion. So it was always, okay, the next time, got to do it the next time. When it started coming back inconclusive, then I knew I blew it. Now we're condoming.

Others recognized that such thinking involved rationalization. Although Ramon ultimately concluded that he had to use condoms, he had not done so for a period of time after he and his wife learned he was positive. "I rationalized it. We've been having intercourse and sex for years and this woman is constantly negative, so the rationale is, hey, I've been doing this for so many years, I don't have to stop doing it. I don't have to use a condom, because nothing's going to happen to her, because if it's going to happen to her it should have happened to her already."

But uninfected individuals permitted themselves to be placed at risk for reasons other than unwillingness to accept that a partner might transmit HIV. To overcome the distance that HIV could create between discordant partners, some had sex without a condom. Paul wanted to feel close to his infected partner, Van, who on occasion urged unsafe sex, as if for one moment to banish the threat of AIDS. "A couple of nights, we didn't use protection," Paul said. "He didn't want to. He said, 'Take this chance one time.' But it could have been a deadly chance. I guess you could say it's luck in a way. I still feel badly because I can't feel what he's feeling, and it hurts me at times to see him suffering, and I speak with God a lot. I say, what can I do? I don't know."

Like uninfected individuals, HIV-positive men and women might also take risks to enhance a sense of intimacy. Emanuel, who was a social worker in an AIDS service organization and was committed to doing "everything right," explained,

> There have been one or two times that we've not used a condom. We talked about it, and it seemed like it was more than passion, because we've had passion so many times. But it seemed like we just wanted to feel closer to each other, to have more from each other, and the condom was in the way. I felt bad, like I should have had more control, and I knew better, and she knew better. I didn't really kick myself in the ass so much for those times, because I think, all things considered, for the amount of time we've been together we've been doing pretty good. I give myself a high rating. Her too. And it wasn't like I came in her or anything like that. I mean, I know about pre-cum and all that. I just wanted to feel that closeness. Because we've been together for six or seven years and never felt each other that way. It's always the condom. It wasn't like if we had started that way, then used condoms, at least we'd have that.

Clearly, protecting partners represents an unending and difficult struggle.

Willingness of uninfected individuals to have unprotected sex with infected partners could also reflect darker motivations, including self-destructive impulses and the thrill of toying with danger. Infected partners then had to decide whether to accede to such needs in a partner. As Christopher, the gay actor, said,

> Even when I have sex with my lover now, I think, God, I love this person so much that if he's negative he could be staying negative, and I'm positive and we're having unsafe sex sometimes. We have a kind of agreement between us that's ours. It's kind of like a wedding ring: we don't care. It's not that we don't care, we just don't stop, we're just so in love with each other. And maybe we should. It's kind of something to think about. Sometimes I really feel guilty and get this mental trip on myself by thinking: if he was ever to get

sick, I would blame me. One time when me and him were first starting to get together his best friend told me, you should tell him to get tested and if he's negative you should break up with him. I mentioned it to my boyfriend and he's like, "Knock it off. I've been doing this same thing before I met you. So it's not you. If I have AIDS, it's not because of you, it's because I've been nuts all my life." I think part of sex is that it's risky, and it's just taking that risk, like it's almost taboo, and then doing the taboo is even more mentally exciting— something that society says is wrong, or is risky. So it's almost even fun. It's like a kid smoking a cigarette behind his momma's back.

It does bother me that he says knock it off. Because I just sometimes think that he has it out for himself. Sometimes I feel like we're both self-destructive. Me and him went through a drug period. Sometimes I feel this is such a self-destructive relationship. We both want to kill ourselves, and I always thought he blamed himself for his lover's death. Like he wasn't there and he's still punishing himself for it. And I'm blaming myself for every other little thing that can come up, like my AIDS. Him going through the whole period of putting a lover in his grave, and now knowing me. I think it scares him. Like, "I don't want to go through this again." When I was in the hospital two weeks ago, it was really hard for him.

Others justified occasional unsafe sex by seeing it as inadvertent and the exception rather than the norm. Claudio, the drug counselor, saw himself as conscientious and committed to his recovery from drug use. He justified having unprotected intercourse, saying that he *usually* withdrew before ejaculating. "I would say 98 percent of the time I practice safer sex, and there've been occasions we have had sex without condoms—mainly oral sex. Intercourse, there's been that on occasion, too. But as a professional I know that's not safe."

Drug use also fostered recklessness. Connie, who had been so drug involved that she was all but oblivious to her pregnancy, gave birth to a "crack baby" who subsequently died. She described how concerns about safety evaporated when she and her uninfected husband were high.

I've told him that I have the virus, but he still won't use condoms. And I told him that I'd rather him use condoms because I don't want him to get sick. But he just doesn't put them on. It hurts because I don't want him to get sick, I really don't. I love him and he's got nine kids of his own. I have one child, and altogether that's ten. Personally, I don't even enjoy sex if I'm getting high. And he knows that, so once in a blue moon he'll bother me about giving him some while he's getting high. I already told him he is going to get infected as long as he is messing with me and I'm infected. I told him point blank, "Walter, I love you. I don't want you to get sick. You know you're supposed to be using a condom. Our counselor told us that when I'm in my menstruation that's the worst time, and that's when you really should use it." He does not do it. I'm not going to sit up there and fuss with him.

Most striking was how the availability of condoms mattered little to her partner.

I get condoms from the clinic each time I'm there. They're all over the place. Closets, everywhere. They get opened. I lay them out and after the high is gone, I sit up there and I'll open up the condoms, I blow them up, tie a knot in them, put them all on the bed. Then when he wakes up the next morning he says, "You had a party here last night." I'll just take a safety pin and pop each one of them.

Condom distribution efforts, however important, were clearly just the beginning of the story.

Though some—particularly women, such as Connie—felt powerless to negotiate protected sex with their partners, others did not appear concerned that having unprotected sex could place a lover at risk. Sexual drive and passion could impel individuals to expose themselves or others to infection. As Neil, the closeted Southerner, said, "Sex makes people do dumb things." Eddie, the current crack and injecting-drug user who eventually infected his wife, said,

When she first got tested she was negative, so then the only proper thing for us to do was to practice safe sex. Sometimes when you get into the heat of the sexual encounters, you don't have condoms, you forget about them. It was like a spur of the moment thing. We had no condoms, and that's when it happened, when we started doing it without it. Not only that but I was uncomfortable with the condoms. I didn't get no feeling from it, and she wasn't too happy with it either. And then they're not always foolproof. It may burst on you or something like that. So we just said, look, hey, we just be careful, and try to withdraw before coming, but you know how you get in the heat of things, sometimes you just can't get out in time.

The worst part came when she became positive. She cried. She got very upset. She was angry so she threw a couple of things in my face: "You could have worn a condom." I said, "Yeah, well you could have made sure I wore one." We did a little verbal whatever at each other. Then after that we calmed down.

She said, "You did this to me. I must love you a hell of a lot to stoop myself to this." Which is true, you know? I don't know if you want to call it a love thing or whatever, but she felt that she loved me more than enough, because she subjected herself to this. So I told her, "I'm sorry," there wasn't much more I could do, "forgive me." I feel bad about it. I know she'd like to punch me in my mouth about twenty-five times for not doing it. But it's been five or six years, and I guess the initial shock is over now. And it's been a healthy relationship since. We are trying to practice safe sex now. We don't do it that much as we used to. Every other time we practice safe sex. We just get involved. I know this is going to sound crazy, but a lot of times we just try to do it, we leave our clothes on and we just like hump and maybe I'll come to a climax, maybe just by the friction. But then when it starts getting too good, then what happens after that, I want to enter and then the condom is forgotten about, because who's going to run to the drawer to get a condom?

This unadorned account illustrates the disjunction between sexual desire and knowledge of what is necessary to prevent HIV transmission—the tension between the "rules" of safe sex and impulse, between selfish gratification and the capacity for and concern about the protection of others. The behavior Eddie continued to engage in was all the more remarkable since he believed that when two infected individuals had unprotected sex they placed themselves at increased risk.

Personally, practicing unsafe sex even if both partners are infected was stupid. Because it's just getting more AIDS, and that doesn't make any sense. The worst part about it is it's not doing nothing to the man, it's more or less doing something to the woman, because the semen is going in, and you're killing her faster, I believe. So you should still practice safe sex regardless if you both are positive. I feel that way.

The disregard for his wife's well-being was underscored by his understanding of a well-established scientific observation—that men can infect women more readily. Thus, he went on, "When I'm doing it, I don't give a damn. But after the fact, I think about it and I say, 'Damn, we should have.' But we didn't. She gets angry about it. She says, 'You should have,' and I says, 'Yeah, I know I should have,' but we didn't. So it was just a Catch-22."

Whatever his regrets, Eddie believed that there were advantages to having an infected wife. "By both of us having it, we come to better terms, we can talk easy. If she didn't have it, she might want to leave me."

Having Children

Individuals knowingly have unsafe sex in another context as well: when a heterosexual couple wants to have children and one member is infected.

Couples in this situation agonize over their choices. During unprotected sexual intercourse, an infected male could infect not only his female partner but, through her, their unborn child as well. When some of these men and women were initially considering the issue, the risk of mother-to-child transmission was widely assumed to be about 20 to 25 percent. In 1994 a clinical trial produced remarkable findings: treatment of infected pregnant women with the antiretroviral drug AZT could reduce the risk to 8 percent.[1] But even this degree of risk of a fatal disease in a child could not be dismissed as utterly insignificant. Couples resolved these decisions in widely differing manners.

One partner's desire to have children could in fact precipitate disclosure. Fred, who had experimented with homosexual encounters while younger and got infected, said,

> It was right before we moved in together. We were planning it, and I sat her down one night and we had this very long discussion. I had told her I had a problem with having children, and she goes, "What, what, what?" She starts rambling out all these different things, and I paused for a little bit and then she blurted out, "AIDS." And I said, "Well I don't exactly have AIDS, but I am HIV positive," and she's crying hysterical, asking questions for about an hour, and we had a long, long talk about it, and I explained to her the parameters, and said, yes, we can get married, but more likely than not we can never have children of our own—my understanding at the time. She said she had to think about it. We talked longer, for several hours, and then the next day she said that she'd go on to move in with me.

Many men struggled with these dilemmas, though concluding that the risks of fathering a child were too great. Frank, the former injecting-drug user who had been a law student, and his wife, who was a social worker, knew of the medically sophisticated options available and had the financial resources to access them.

> Initially she was more interested in it, and my reaction was, "What, are you crazy? You can't do that." And she said, "Other babies are born with HIV and they don't die right away." But I'd say within a month or two she got over that. I guess she couldn't deal with the trauma of being told she couldn't do it, so she was looking for a way out.
>
> Last year we did seven months of artificial insemination with a donor, with supposedly one of the top experts here in the city, and it didn't work. She wants to continue. It's been a couple of months, and I changed my mind near the end, in the sixth month or so, and she went ahead and did a seventh

month without my approval. And now we're in negotiation about doing it again, for another course of treatment. I'm leaning toward not wanting to do it. But I feel confused about it. I'm afraid of the consequences of having a baby, considering what might happen to me and my current situation, financially, healthwise, emotionally. The other side of the coin is that it's extremely important to my wife and it's difficult for me to refuse her. Also, as a lot of people have suggested to me, it may be very good for me. It may help me enjoy life more, give me new sustenance. And they may be right. It's hard for me really to sort it all out and make a decision. But I'm fearful of it not working well.

I've thought a little bit about the sperm washing that they're doing at the University of Milan. They seem to have had a lot of success there, but I'm not quite sure. It's overwhelming, dealing with all of this, not just emotionally, but there's just so much to deal with that I'm having trouble now taking sufficient interest to call Milan to investigate it. I understand they've had a number of participants, about thirty, and they've never transmitted the virus, and they've had a pretty good success rate with pregnancy. But I'm worried about my DNA. I've been using AZT for two years. I'm worried maybe I couldn't have a healthy child no matter what, so I really have to investigate that.

In raising the issue of a genetic threat to his potential child (a concern without scientific merit), Frank in part intimated a more basic fear: the prospect that his child, even if healthy, could be fatherless.

In this and other instances, couples confronting questions of childbearing had to weigh dreams, hopes, and fears. Conflict often resulted as partners differed about the acceptability of risk. Where one partner might see a chance worth taking, the other might see too great a gamble with life. Fred's uninfected wife had delivered a healthy child, but he was reluctant to try having a second child. Of note, she thought the risk tolerable. Fred stated,

When we found out from a specialist doctor that it is highly unlikely to have an HIV-positive child from an HIV-negative mother, and that one or two exposures are also not likely to be that dangerous, we were very gung ho about it, especially my wife. It's her decision as far as that's concerned, exposing herself. It's completely her decision. In fact she's talking about a second child now, and I've always been backing away from it because the risk is there. I don't like the idea of having an only child. I think that a kid should have a brother or sister. I grew up with a brother and a sister. But it's not worth risking not having a mother. So I've been shying away. She's been pushing. Every time she brings it up, she asks when. I say, well, let's wait a little bit, the spread isn't enough between the kids, wait until one will be in school and the other one's . . . I've been making up bullshit excuses. She's anxious to do it again.

She doesn't think that it'll be a problem, or if it will be a problem, she'll deal with it. But I don't know if I'm ready to.

Other couples resolved the conflicts by temporizing their actions—chancing fate and trying for limited periods of time to have a child. "My T-cell count was very high even though I was positive," said Keith, the former drug user who worked for the phone company, and whose wife was not infected.

> We were racing against a clock, trying to have a kid, and we decided to take the risk having unprotected sex so that she could conceive. And she did. But then she miscarried, and we said, that's it. I have a son and a daughter through my prior marriage, and she has a son through her prior marriage, and that's enough. We both accepted that we're not going to do it.

Despite professional counseling, some chose to take the risk, at least for a time. Ramon said of the period just after he learned he was infected,

> When we started going to the health center, they told my wife that we should never try to have any children. When my wife got pregnant and my son came out healthy, that was a blessing in disguise. We were totally concerned about that, because she knew I was HIV positive and that there was a chance of her converting. And we just rolled the dice and came up seven. So once that had happened, it was, hey, we're lucky, we're fortunate, let's just use these condoms, let's use protection like we're supposed to. Now—having a child, and also being concerned for my wife and her well-being, too—we have to do the mature thing.

In his mind, maturity necessitated safety rather than risk taking.

Some couples repeatedly revisited these difficult decisions. They took into account changing understandings of the clinical course of HIV in children, given improvements in therapy and, most importantly, the prospects for reducing the risk of mother-to-child transmission. Jane, whose husband was HIV negative, very much wanted to have a child, but in the end couldn't face the consequences.

> We decided to adopt. Then we decided we didn't want to adopt, but wanted me to get pregnant, that we would take the 25 or 30 percent chance I'd have an infected baby—and live with the consequences of it. If we were willing to love the child and care for it, then we should go ahead and do it. Then I started getting uncomfortable with that and thinking about what would happen if the baby were sick and how would I feel.

Yet even after AZT was found to reduce radically the risk of having an infected child, Jane could not accept the prospect of bearing a child with HIV infection. "Now it's down to 8 percent, and I still couldn't live with it."

Negotiated Safety

Couples in which both members test negative can also decide not to use condoms, a choice termed "negotiated safety" by its advocates. Others deride such a choice, seeing it as too risky, because one partner might "import" HIV to the relationship. Some critics, noting the extent to which monogamy is uncommon among gay couples, have dubbed such decisions "negotiated danger." Why would people embrace a possibly lethal course?

Partners may have complete and utter faith in the principle of mutual trust. Before his current relationship, David, the teachers' union official, had been extremely cautious about what he would risk doing. But now, given that he and his current lover were both negative, they decided not to use condoms. "My sex with my lover is almost all anal. I'm passive, he's active. We don't use condoms: I trust him. That's the best way to put it. I have a feeling he's not cheating. I could be wrong, of course." He acknowledged that "in a way" he was putting his life in his partner's hands. "And in a way he is with me, too, for that matter. I feel that if he were going to cheat, he would tell me. As I would tell him." He assessed how his age—he was 61—might make such a choice more reasonable. "I think if I were 30 or 35, I might always practice safe sex. I would probably be tempted myself, as I would presume he would be, too."

Such trust could be total, almost sacrosanct. As Otis, the uninfected social worker, revealed, it was as if AIDS did not exist.

> My lover and I were together two years and we both were tested together, and were negative. We were in a relationship together, and there was a lot of love there. He was a lover. He broke up with me for various reasons, but he's someone I really wish I was still with, and I was in love with him, so everything was open, total. It was as if AIDS never existed between us. We were about as low risk as could be, even though we were both out gay men in New York City in 1991. We did everything. We were monogamous, and there was total trust. I don't fool around with that, and he didn't either. No, never. And ultimately what happened in the relationship, he told me that he did play around a few times where he traveled on business or whatever, but what he had done was totally safe. In other words he didn't get fucked, he didn't fuck.
>
> We did fuck. That was something that was extremely special; I mean, he

was somebody I really loved, really enjoyed sexually. The Ideal Lover. I put all my trust, all my energies into that.

Heterosexual couples, among whom monogamy was the norm, commonly eschewed condoms when both partners tested negative. Gloria, who had lived in a crack house, felt her deepening relationship with her husband made condoms unnecessary. "When I first met Colin, he used a condom, but we stopped. We drew closer to each other, more confident, more secure. I knew my situation, he knew his, and he felt that if I did anything, if he had anything, he wouldn't have hurt me."

Similarly, other couples decided to stop using condoms at some point in the evolution of their relationship. Nancy, the former textile designer infected by a boyfriend, said, "I've heard a lot of people say that at first they use condoms and then they start to feel comfortable and trust this person, and lose the condoms somewhere along the way." But uncertainty could haunt such decisions. When could a partner finally be trusted? How certain could one be of the promise of fidelity? The price of error was high.

Those who took the chance typically assumed that they could detect if a partner cheated and violated the trust necessary for such unprotected sex. Although her risks from sex with her lesbian partners were small, Carla, uninfected, was nevertheless concerned. She or her partner could become infected by trading sex with men for drugs or money. "If it's monogamous and you think it's okay to have unprotected sex, you would just have to have trust. If you got to know the person you could pretty much tell when somebody's cheating. It's just the attitude or something, most people can tell when somebody's cheating." But were such assumptions little more than wishful thinking? Love may be total, but blind; some who fully trusted partners nonetheless became infected.

Conversely, to begin using condoms in an established relationship could stir distrust. Audrey, the infected sociology student whose husband was not infected, said,

> On the one hand, I would say everybody should use condoms no matter what, and on the other hand, you have to balance that against introducing mistrust into a long-term, possibly stable, wonderful relationship, and you know what harm that can introduce. So it's a really tough issue. I think definitely people in monogamous relationships should get tested together, and beyond that I don't know. If you've both been tested and you both find out you're negative, and then you say, look I still want to use condoms even though we have this other acceptable method of birth control that worked

fine for us before, it's obviously because I don't trust you or I'm fucking around. It's an issue: mistrust.

Hidden Dangers: Unsafe Sex without Disclosure

Some infected individuals did not disclose to partners before having unsafe sex. Such failures to disclose raise very different moral, social, and psychological issues than when an infected individual has unsafe sex with a consenting partner who is fully aware of the risks of HIV transmission or when an individual fails to disclose but engages in "safer sex." Our interviews indicated that unsafe sex without disclosure occurred for a variety of social, cultural, and psychological and moral reasons. In some instances, norms within different subcultures made such acts acceptable. Denial about the extent to which one posed a lethal threat to others played a role, too. Finally, destructive anger or indifference to others' needs could also fuel such behavior.

Particular settings can sanction and even facilitate unprotected sex without disclosure. As we noted earlier in our discussion of disclosure in sex clubs and bathhouses, setting and context shape norms and expectations. The riskiness of encounters in these sex-charged environments might in fact augment the sense of excitement. Although there is considerable dispute about the extent to which those who frequent bathhouses and sex clubs use condoms, a number of the men with whom we spoke described participating in or witnessing unsafe sex. As Lance, the gay man who suggested that silence in bathhouses was an "unspoken" rule, explained, "People are not going to use safe sex in those arenas, because it's uncomfortable, and there's a certain element of risk in it that you find attractive."

Bathhouses could represent a kind of escape, permitting dangerous acts that would otherwise be unacceptable. Though he spoke of the values of twelve-step programs and believed that self-honesty was indispensable to his own sobriety, Lance continued,

> The bathhouses are kind of a sanity. You shut out the outside world, and for me especially that was true. You could live out your fantasies, and in your fantasies HIV doesn't exist, and everybody's beautiful and having sex, whatever kind of sex it is that you subscribe to, and reality just doesn't sink in, unfortunately. I mean, people are using safe sex at the bathhouses, but I think one of the things that has to be remembered, too, is that a lot of the people that go to the bathhouses are high, and when you're high, on whatever substance, you're less likely to take precautions. It's just immediate gratification. I think that has a lot to do with it.

In fact, with improved treatments for HIV, such behavior might have increased. As Christopher, the actor who had been a hustler, suggested, while sex clubs waned following the beginning of the HIV epidemic, they burgeoned in the mid-1990s.

> There's tons of sex clubs now. I know guys that are HIV positive that go to those sex clubs three nights a week and don't use condoms or nothing like that. They go into the back room and party up. There's a big rampant sexual thing going on right now. The sex clubs and the sex and the drugs, that whole thing is happening right now, again, like the '70s almost.

Many sought such settings to connect to others through sex, minimizing the risks taken or imposed. As George, the psychologist, said, eight years after his HIV diagnosis, "In the baths and clubs people are still engaging in unsafe sex. I think it's about the power of sex and the need to connect."

Others rationalized as well that they had no moral responsibility toward partners willing to engage in unsafe sex. Ben, who was infected, said,

> I have at various locations believed that people must be aware of the fact that many other people present were likely to be HIV carriers, infected, and assumed that if there is a million in one chance of contracting the illness by unprotected fellatio, for example, that they're there voluntarily, and I have not felt any particular moral qualms about participating to the extent of having fellatio performed, certainly without getting close to ejaculation.

He sought to temper his account by noting that he exercised some restraint by not ejaculating. He also emphasized the absence of responsibility for what occurred by stressing that what he gave, his partners were free to reject. But then he went on to say, "Occasionally—this is getting into a murky area—I'll meet a partner who is into water sports, and I have pissed on someone, and it may have splashed onto their tongue. I may equate that with giving someone a carton of cigarettes for a gift. There's certainly some risk, but also there's some pleasure." He saw his freedom to act as morally equivalent to the freedom of others to choose and to make their own risk-benefit calculations. It was a moral world in which "let the buyer beware" served as a guiding rule.

Questions arose as to whether such behaviors could or should be controlled in these environments. Despite the efforts to reduce such practices through monitors, unsafe sex could persist. Sam, the respiratory therapist, observed,

> I know that they have sex police in some of these backroom after-hours places, where they keep you from being unsafe. I think unfortunately it's nec-

essary, because some people may drink too much and get wildly out of control. I mean, it's kind of like the state's controlling your sex, but the goal here I
think is to stop the infection with the virus. And if it takes them shining flash-
lights on people in dark rooms, then that's great.

Others, including civil libertarians, most AIDS activists, and many public
health officials, are skeptical about the benefit of restrictive public health
measures. Craig, the former male prostitute, cautioned against the effectiveness of trying to impose restrictions in such settings.

It's not the location. If a person's going to have unsafe sex, they're gonna do it
behind closed doors or in a public place or a public forum. You can shut down
every sex club on this island, they're still going to be in the bushes in Central
Park. There are many places in the city. It's not going to stop anything by shut-
ting down, and even the sleaziest sex clubs do provide condoms and lubrica-
tion. It is the individual that chooses to go into those places. I think basically
everyone is aware of the safe sex thing, and there are people that choose not
to have safe sex, to blatantly swallow a load, fully aware I'm sure, unless
they've been in a cave for the past few years, of what's going on.

Unsafe sex occurs not only in anonymous encounters for sexual pleasure
but also among those who exchange sex for money or drugs. In this context,
as described earlier, disclosure rarely occurs—it is simply not part of the commercial norm. Pam, who was infected, said that if she disclosed to customers
she would lose business. "They'd say, 'See ya.'" As a result, her strategy was to
"spit cum out of my mouth." By emphasizing what she did to protect herself,
she clearly thought that as a sex worker she had no obligation to her clients.
As noted earlier, those who bought sex often seemed unconcerned about the
possibility that sex workers might be infected.

According to our interviewees, infected clients never disclosed to sex
workers and typically insisted that their sexual encounters occur without
condoms, compelling commercial sex workers to take whatever measures
seemed appropriate or possible. Although many sought to protect themselves with condoms, others took the risks necessary to get the money they
needed. Beatrice, who had managed to remain uninfected, suggested the
precarious struggle between danger from HIV and the need for drugs or
money.

I was out there because I wanted drugs. Now with a couple of them, I would
say, "Will you use this?" And if he said, "No," I said, "Well I got to look, study,
see if you got any bumps, open sores." But later when it came to AIDS and I
was out there, I just was too scared, because I seen so many die of this stuff, so

> I would say, "Well if you don't want it, somebody else will. Use this or no." I want to get high, but not my life, no. I got a little pride in me, that's why I never went too low in the gutter, 'cause I always thought a little bit more of myself than that. Yes, I was using drugs; yes, I was turning tricks. But one day I was going to stop all of this, I always looked to the future, that I was going to stop, and I got daughters, so, no, I wasn't into that.

Although she said she now turned down potential clients who might be infected and wouldn't use condoms, she suggested that, in the past, she might have had unsafe sex with someone whose status she felt—but didn't necessarily know—was negative.

Unsafe sex without disclosure occurs not only in settings defined by anonymity, cash, or drugs, where the possibility of HIV transmission is understood, but in relationships—both casual as well as intimate, where assumptions about the presence of risk vary.

As our interviewees have described, the heat of passion could lead to unsafe sex without disclosure even by individuals who thought they *might* be infected. Darryl, for example, who had spent years in jail and was committed to recovering from his drug use, used condoms before his diagnosis but nevertheless placed his girlfriend at risk. "What went through my head was, damn, just suppose I am infected, I'd be putting her at risk. But I guess in the heat of passion—a lot of time it overrides intellectual thinking."

Others knew they were positive but engaged in unsafe sex without disclosure. Some did so assuming that no additional risk existed for them, that their partners were in all likelihood already infected. Gary said,

> I never left home without my rubbers. These days, I think I'm joining a majority of positive people who, when you're with somebody positive it's like, what, are you going to catch something? I know you can logically. But it's nice to have sex without a condom and not be worried. It's just more intimate. So that's where I'm at right now. Occasionally I use them, but not that much.

When asked if he had had sex with anyone who was negative, he responded, "No. I never run into people that are negative."

Rationalizations, even self-acknowledged, could abet such risky behavior, minimizing appraisals of the dangers involved. Patrick, the closeted bisexual police officer, ultimately took two years to tell the woman he loved and would marry about his HIV infection. In that period he continued to have unprotected sex with her. He also did not disclose to casual sexual partners with whom he had unprotected intercourse, though withdrawing before ejaculation.

There were three women, prior to my wife, that were one-night stands. I can remember thinking that as long as I don't come in them—and now I know that's totally fucking false—but my thinking was, well, just don't come in them. I always pulled out toward the end. I thought about it, but a lot of lust was there, driving me toward just having sex. There was concern, but not enough at that time to make me stop, or think of using a condom, because I just didn't. Now I carry contraceptives, but then it was not a thing.

Moral awareness thus provided a poor antidote to sexual desire.

In some instances, unsafe sex without disclosure could result from feelings of loneliness, stigma, and rejection and could lead to remorse. Remarkably, some were concerned mostly with how they might have placed themselves at risk. For example, Lance, who was infected and now a recovering alcoholic, said,

I guess I was trying to hurt myself, too. It was anonymous sex. I was the receptive partner and he did not use a condom. Nothing was said. I guess I was sort of desperate: I needed the validation. And I felt very guilty afterward about what the consequences of it could have been. So far, nothing's showed up, but still it was very foolish, I felt very guilty about it for days afterward. That I could have hurt myself, that my immune system's very sensitive at this point, and that I don't have the resistance that I would if my immune system wasn't impaired. I thought I had come so far, and to have a relapse disappointed me. Loneliness, I think, had a lot to do with it. I remember when I had a bad acid trip, one of my greatest fears was that no one was ever going to be able to love me, and it was so intense, it was like a physical pain. And the anonymous sex was kind of like that, except not as intense, because the drugs weren't involved. Just being so desperately alone. To me it seems even if you're in a relationship, you're still alone to a certain extent, and once my relationship with my lover broke up, it left me at loose ends and brought that feeling back again of being desperate and lonely. It was a momentary satisfaction.

Indifference to the well-being of others—due in part to drugs—could also lead to nondisclosure and unsafe sex. Though adopting more responsible behavior in recent years, Dolores, the "black sheep" in her family, described how while hustling in the street she had ignored the risks she could pose to partners who were not customers.

I probably slept with people and didn't tell them neither, because at that time I didn't care. Now it's a whole new thing for me, it's something I did to myself, nobody did this to me. Why make somebody else's life miserable because I did something to me? But back then if I wasn't married and had a partner to sleep with every day at my own house, I probably would sleep with anybody—didn't make no difference. I was drugging, too.

Much of the AIDS-prevention effort has, for obvious reasons of public health, emphasized the importance of practicing safer sex—that is, using condoms. Indeed, these efforts have prioritized safer sex over disclosure. Yet in these interviews we have discovered how, for a variety of reasons—related to intimacy, the courting of danger, and the desire to bear children—individuals, even after disclosure, elected to eschew condoms. Such choices were made both by infected men and women who could transmit HIV and by uninfected individuals who could place themselves at risk. No understanding of the dynamics of living with HIV would be complete without an appreciation of how and why such decisions are made. Nor could an understanding of moral issues posed by dangerous intimacies be complete without an appreciation of the complex relationship between the assumption—the taking on—of risk and the freedom to choose.

Finally, as we have seen in the discussion of hidden dangers, others chose to engage in unsafe sex without disclosure. Those who encountered such individuals in venues known to be hazardous could choose to protect themselves. In other circumstances, trust or naïveté made condoms seem unnecessary, though dangers hovered. The only "protection" was that exposure did not always result in transmission. Here, the moral issues seem clear. But as we shall see, questions remain far from settled as to how to respond to individuals who willingly endanger others.

6 | MAKING MORAL JUDGMENTS

In communities where HIV-related suffering, disease, and death were widespread, men and women—both infected and uninfected—inevitably had to confront questions of whether and how to judge those who placed others at risk. Many of the individuals we interviewed saw no alternative but to assign blame where they thought it was due. Yet others resisted the lure or pressure to pass moral judgment on individuals, seeing in the intimate nature of HIV transmission private matters beyond moral critique.

The Question of Blame

Almost invariably, those who had been infected had to wrestle with questions of the extent to which they had made themselves vulnerable and bore some responsibility for acquiring the virus. Many knew how they had been exposed—years of drug use and the sharing of injection equipment; prostitution; a series of sexual encounters (heterosexual or homosexual), some of which might have been anonymous. Such cumulative risk precluded the assignment of blame, which seemed beside the point. Nancy, the former textile designer, was diagnosed while hospitalized with PCP. Her boyfriend was also infected, and she believed she had unknowingly infected him.

> I'd slept around when I was younger. In the early '80s, one guy left me for a guy. I didn't know about AIDS then. When I was 22 years old I slept with a person who was an IV drug user, who swore he'd been tested. My mother just keeps wanting to know where I got it from, and I keep telling her I don't know. That really infuriates her. She can't blame somebody else. Even if I did know where I got it, I don't know if I'd tell her. Because of the blame thing, I don't think I would. I don't think it's right.

Some could neither blame their sexual partners nor tolerate the thought that they had placed themselves at risk. Peter, the young married doctor who spoke only reluctantly of homosexual encounters in the past, said, "I had one or two homosexual encounters, just an experimental type of thing," though he went on to describe a relationship that lasted "one or two months."

> We'd just get together from time to time and drink, and had a couple of sexual encounters after that. I found out later on, about two years ago, he died of AIDS. It was very upsetting. I had had sex with this guy, and after the summer we just sort of lost contact with each other, lost a sense of friendship, and then hadn't heard from him or about him in five, six years. Then to read about it in the college bulletin was a very big shock. I don't think it's anybody's fault; it isn't really all that important, as compared to the fact that now you're infected, now you have to deal with it. I could spend the entire rest of my life agonizing over, "Was it so-and-so, or this or that event?" But it's not going to change anything. It can't change the course. I have to put that behind me. Otherwise I can't go on with my own life.

Even those who wanted to know the source of their infection commonly faced uncertainty. As one woman said, "The only way I can figure I got it was either through my son's father—we broke up in 1983—or the man I was with before my husband. He says that he doesn't have it. But I don't know how much to believe him." Chuck, the gay man living in a shelter, thought he was infected by a male partner who previously had dated a drag queen. When asked whether either of these other individuals had the virus, he answered, "No. No. Not 'fact fact.' I don't know by fact. But I believe he had it. He's still living, but the drag queen died." Like others, he had no surety, only suspicions.

Betrayals of Trust

A number of men and women felt certain about the source of their infection and wrestled with feelings of betrayal. Some were infected by casual partners, others in ongoing relationships. In either case, those who had been infected had to confront the question of whether they had been deceived, whether the risk of HIV had been masked, and whether their trust and love had been abused.

Some sought to deal with betrayal by protecting the relationship, grasping at the possibility that they had not been willfully harmed by their partners. Diagnosed at 34, Regina, whose 7-year-old son died of AIDS, said of her former lover,

> He knew something was wrong because he kept telling me he didn't think he'd live to be 35. I don't think he knew specifically it had anything to do with

the AIDS. But he had a feeling something wasn't right. He's never even ad-
mitted going and getting tested. I don't know if he ever did. I don't think he
knew. I don't even want to believe that he had an idea something like that was
wrong. Because to have known that, he would have known that he was playing with not only his life, he was playing Russian roulette with mine also.

Many made a conscious decision to eschew accusation and blame, to protect both the individual who might have infected them and the relationship
within which the transmission might have occurred. The transmission of
HIV was a tragedy, not a misdeed. Maria, the secretary, was 27 when a former
boyfriend notified her that he had AIDS. "When we were together we really
loved each other," she said. "If it happened, it wasn't intentional. I wasn't
angry." Indeed it was characteristic of her that she said she felt "gratitude" to
him for informing her, because "I wouldn't be considering myself one of the
high-risk groups."

Yet some blamed their partners as being irresponsible in practicing unsafe
sex. Despite the prevailing recommendation to use condoms in every sexual
encounter, Maurice, who thought he could assess others' trustworthiness
based on his experience as a teacher, had trusted his lover and thus exposed
himself to HIV.

Since I tested negative and then six months later was HIV positive, I was infected during that six months period. I was seeing only one person during
that six-month period—my lover—who insisted that he had not been tested,
but that there was no way that he could be positive. Then it turns out, when
he gets tested after me, that he's positive. It was somewhat irresponsible on
his part to be so sure that he couldn't be positive. Because he said that he had
to be negative. I basically assumed that that meant he had practiced safe sex.
I don't think we would have been as unsafe as we were if I had reason to think
that he might be positive.

He explained that this partner "loved me as intensely as anybody has ever
loved me in my life. He didn't do it consciously. Whatever happened it was
either because he was in denial or didn't really understand. He didn't at that
time realize the ways in which he might have been exposed." Maurice's
struggle to understand what had happened to him thus entailed both a judgment, "he was responsible," and an effort at exculpation, "he didn't do it
consciously." Thus, Maurice sought to balance his anger with his need to
protect his understanding of both the man he loved and their relationship.
Here, too, questions arise about the degree to which individuals can be held
morally accountable when deceiving themselves.

When HIV transmission occurred in an intimate relationship in which the infected partner had consciously hidden the truth—about either the presence or the risk of HIV—despair and outrage amplified the sense of betrayal. Confusion and bewilderment could ensue. Only with difficulty did Audrey, the Ph.D. candidate diagnosed in her early twenties, come to see that her ex-boyfriend, Julio, did not disclose his risky behaviors—sharing needles—or, after they broke up, knowledge of his infection.

> We had had conversations about it, but I guess we either didn't think it was real enough to get tested for, or we were too scared. But I wonder now—and I have no idea if I'm totally imagining this—if he knew he could have been infecting me, that maybe he was trying already to set the seeds, or blame it on somebody else. Because I definitely went into the testing situation thinking it could have only been another guy. I had no clue that Julio could have done it, and it wasn't until after I called Julio and told him I was positive—that was a tough one, too—that I really started to question, that I realized he was lying to me.
>
> When I called and told him I was infected, he was like, "Oh, poor baby, poor baby," and I'm like, "Well what about you? You've got to get tested." And he's like, "Oh, my God I'm sure I have it, I'm sure I have it." I'm like, "Oh, no, you don't know, it's hard for women to transmit it to men, just get tested, and we'll find out." And he's like, "No, I'm certain I am, I'm certain I am," which is logical, I mean, anybody would feel like that. But he's like, "Oh, I had shingles in March." And that is the thing that really fucking killed me: that he should have known when he had shingles. I mean denial, fine, but at that point there's no reason for denial any more. And what really kills me about that is that I was still sleeping with Bill, my boyfriend, with no protection. I just thank God Bill was not infected in that time. Yet I was still being really stupid. When Julio told me about having shingles in that conversation, I'm like, "Oh, well, you know, sometimes adults have that." I was trying to reassure him. I guess he called me a few weeks later and told me that his came back positive.

Ultimately, she believed he had deceived her about the extent to which he had placed her at risk, because he had not made clear that he himself was at risk.

> I think he lied, but I just don't know where the lie is. I don't know if he lied about being tested, or maybe he was sharing needles after he was tested. But I'm very convinced that he did infect me. I don't think he knew that he was infected. I think he just knew he was at risk and was kind of trying to bury the idea. I would say that people should be able to have a feeling as to whether or not there's something like that going on in the relationship, but I had no clue

that I could not trust Julio. I got this because somebody lied to me and I feel very indignant: I did all the right things and still this happened to me.

Falsehood could also be more explicit and, in retrospect, more clear. When Gladys, the telephone company manager, was diagnosed with HIV, she felt starkly betrayed, robbed of her life.

> When I learned he had AIDS, that didn't bother me as much as that he didn't tell me. We had been together six years. Of course, condoms after a while went by the wayside. It was a monogamous relationship, so I had no fears about it. He had been hospitalized twice before with pneumonia; he had informed me that it was not PCP, the pneumonia that affects those with HIV. I just didn't think he would lie to me about it. Because we had discussed it several times prior, because he's an ex-IV drug user. I thought we could be open and honest. But he couldn't handle it that way. I just can't imagine that he would put me in that position, jeopardize my life like that. That's what's so painful: "I thought you loved me." I was devastated because he knew and didn't tell me. I trusted him. I was just angry. I just wanted to know, "Why? Why didn't you tell me, what were you trying to do? I thought we were getting married, that you loved me, why didn't you tell me?" He went to the grave with that. I never found out.

Despite her outrage, her love for the man she had planned to marry permitted her to be at his side in the last stages of his disease, to support him as he lay dying. She was able to do so by assuming some of the responsibility for her own infection.

> I blame me more so than him, but it's easier to be angry with him. I should have known better. I mean, his history was there that he was an ex-IV drug user. But then I trusted, and I am angry at myself. This is the first time I ever trusted a man to that extent, and I just should have known. But I just didn't see it, because I just didn't want to think that he would put me in that position and not say anything. Sometimes I beat myself up so bad. It's very hard. He's not the only one to blame, it's just that I feel so ridiculous. I've come along so far, raising three children and working—and this? That's why I say I feel ridiculous, because I know better. I trusted someone who betrayed me. And I know better than to trust someone, but then I say, you got to trust somebody. I try to make it so that I can understand, but I don't.

Dishonesty like that encountered by Gladys could be even more explicit. Jane, who had been tested when she and her husband wanted to have children, said,

I actually know a woman like that. Her husband was taking AZT, and when she said to him, "What is this?" he said, "It's for part of my rehab." She was finally infected, and confronted him, and he said, "Oh, yeah." He did know all along. I have never thought something like that was possible. But then you hear about battered women and about other types of abusive relationships. I guess that's what it is, it's an abusive relationship. In this case it's even more deadly, being infected with a fatal illness.

Lies could also be part of a larger plan of cunning, deception, and harm. Jennifer, the computer graphics designer, certain she had no reason to believe she was at risk for AIDS, discovered her HIV infection as the result of donating blood. Speaking of the man who had infected her, she bitterly recalled,

He just seemed to be the most perfect guy. Anything I wanted, anything that I was interested in, anywhere I wanted to go. He was sweet and loving and just all those things you really don't find in too many guys anymore, and he turned out to be a liar. I went back to him and told him that I was HIV positive and that I thought that he should get himself checked out, and he was devastated. But as it turns out, he knew, not only that he was HIV positive, he really had full-blown AIDS, and he had deceived me in that. It turns out he was just a cad and a scoundrel. Later he told me he knowingly infected me, that he had picked me out and he found out a lot about me, and that he wanted me to be his mate for life. Who else would have him? If he infected me, then who else would have me but somebody like him. So he purposely destroyed my life. I believe people, or I did believe people, and I trusted unconditionally. He must have picked up on that, and he just took a deer and threw a grenade at it. He's evil. He is evil. I believe he is evil. He's a sick fuck.

The accounts of both Gladys and Jennifer suggest that greater vigilance might have identified potentially life-saving warning signs. That they had been deceived and that they had deceived themselves is clear. But the moral issues entailed here highlight the profound differences between these types of deception. The deception to which each woman had been subjected—by men who had put them at risk—was very different from the self-deception that had opened them to danger. At most, Gladys and Jennifer had been foolish. Their male partners had behaved malignantly.

Resisting Moral Judgments

Individuals had to confront questions of guilt, blame, and responsibility concerning not only their own and their partners' behavior but often, too, that of friends and acquaintances. Not uncommonly, our interviewees knew of men and women, either directly or by report, whose actions placed others at risk. Individuals aware of such hazardous behavior reacted based on a range of factors—whether or not they were infected, how they viewed their responsibilities to their own sexual partners, whether they believed they had the ability to protect themselves, and how close they felt to those put at risk. As they came to grips with these matters, men and women commonly sought and employed metaphors and analogies to grasp the moral principles at play.

Many found it difficult to pass judgment—even on those who endangered others—as their own past troubles made them acutely aware of how problematic moral assessments could be. That did not mean these individuals saw the world as an amoral place. As Christopher, the gay actor, said about why he could not judge such individuals, "Who am I to judge anybody for not telling anything, because I've done so much shit in my life? I can't judge anybody for doing anything." Nevertheless, he believed that "the universe takes care of its people" and that "something would be done" to those who spread HIV.

The world within which gay men found themselves, and the isolation that had resulted from stigma and ostracism while growing up, could provide both an explanation and exculpation. Speaking about those who had many anonymous sexual encounters, Steve, the uninfected pet store owner who lived with an infected lover, noted,

> For so many gay people, sex is the whole thing. The only place they can find somebody who at least cares for them for an hour is to pick them up. Unfortunately, it's the only thing that they know. If it's between two consenting adults, I don't feel I have any question of stopping it. They're making their own health more imperiled, and they're imperiling others. Nobody's without guilt, everybody's responsible for their own actions.

Stigma and discrimination against gay men could result in particularly desperate situations that in turn could further promote risky behavior. David, the teachers' union official, believed adults had a responsibility to protect their sexual partners, yet understood why some gay adolescents, rejected by their families, could end up jeopardizing themselves and others.

> I saw a kid in school, his father found out that he was seeing another boy and his father came home and found them in bed together. The father threw his son out, saying, "I don't want to see you again." About two months later I was in the city. I saw him hustling, and so I went over to him and said, "What the hell are you doing?" and he said, "This is the only way I can earn a living."

I said, "But you're going to get the disease. You can't turn down a partner or what they're going to do, because you want the money and they're not going to be responsible about telling you that they have the disease." I saw him about a year later and he was infected, and still hustling.

Some refused to judge or confront others for strategic reasons—because such an approach could backfire. While morally troubled by what he saw, Steve believed it crucial to adopt a tone of neutrality.

I work with a guy now who's never been in a relationship and he'll walk home from work and see somebody in Central Park and go under a bridge and have sex with them, and he knows it's not safe. And I say, "What are you doing?" He tells me everything that he's doing. He's having oral sex, anal sex with these people, unprotected, and when I'm asking him what's he doing, I'm asking him what is he doing to himself. He is so alone that any contact is better than no contact. I talk to him about it and ask him if he's being safe, and it's "Well . . ." But he's very concerned about being judged, so I'm trying to get him to comply without me turning around and being judgmental on him, because I know that once it's judgmental, he's just going to shut up and he's got nobody to at least talk to about it.

The philosophy of recovery groups that reject judgmentalism also contributed to such a posture. Darryl, who had entered recovery after many years of drug use, said, "I have a couple of friends and one of them did not practice safe sex after knowing he was positive and infected his wife, and another one refused to use protection with anybody he has sex with. What I normally do is pray to God to please allow me not to judge this person and just accept them as they are."

Those who worked as mental health professionals most fully articulated a stance of neutrality, reflecting what they understood to be the dictates of good clinical practice. Working in a drug-treatment program, Claudio, the infected counselor and former drug user, said about his clients, "I'm an educator and I give them their space. It's their choice. I can't tell them what to do. I don't preach to them, 'You need to do this or you have to do that, or don't you know you're committing a crime.' They're pretty much intelligent and informed people, so they have their conscience. They have their own beliefs."

Those who declined to pass judgment were still often troubled by the implications of what they observed. George, the gay man who trained in psychology after being diagnosed with HIV, described his encounter with a prisoner who had imperiled others.

I remember one telling me that he was pissed off, and he decided he was go-ing to infect as many people as he could. It's hard to hear. I can empathize with his anger at being infected, but . . . He told me a story of running into someone who he infected or said that he infected, and he at least had enough superego that he felt some guilt. I've never been one for coercive measures like quarantine. I certainly wished that he had been able to get some kind of help or find someone to talk to, because I think there are other ways to express anger.

Caveat Emptor

As noted earlier, many believed that in the face of the AIDS epidemic, only an attitude of caveat emptor could be protective. From that vantage point, all individuals were responsible for protecting themselves. The infected had no special duty to safeguard their partners. Many HIV-negative as well as HIV-positive individuals shared this attitude. "I think it's the buyer beware today," said Morris, the uninfected gay man who tolerated the risks of un-protected oral sex with an infected lover. "If you're out there seeking sex, you'd better be aware of what you're doing and with whom you're doing it." He continued, "Everyone has an obligation to protect themselves, and if you choose to have unsafe sex without knowing the status of your partner, that's a risk that you must be willing to take. It takes two people to do this, and I be-lieve in individual responsibility." George, the psychologist, anticipated with hard realism any objections to the stance of caveat emptor. "You have to assume that everybody's HIV positive, because people do lie. If they had no reason to suspect, then that to me is not a very good answer these days. There's always reason to suspect."

Repeatedly, those who were infected drew on justifications they used for their own acts to explain their unwillingness to judge others. Assuming that all partners could pose potential danger, Ben, who was infected and saw himself as an "almost moral man," viewed the risks of sex as analogous to those of the open road. "I think HIV is probably present in most people who are sexually not monogamous, sexually active with more than one partner. A kind of defensive driving, where you assume that everybody is a reckless driver—I think that's the attitude." He went on to minimize the extent of his responsibility toward others by assuming that those who took risks must al-ready be infected.

I have protested being the inserter in unprotected anal sex, with at least one partner, perhaps two, who have insisted that it be unprotected. And with at least one partner I reached orgasm, maybe a couple of years ago. That caused me some pause, but I suppose I concluded that the partner was also in my category and therefore willing to accept the risk.

Others looked to examples of particular individuals to bolster their beliefs. Carl, the infected masseur in an "open" relationship with Gerry, who was uninfected, had acknowledged that in outside liaisons he had unprotected sex "about 25 to 30 percent of the time." For Carl, everyone was ultimately responsible for himself—not for others. "My theory, and actually Gerry's the perfect proof of it, has always been that you have to look out for yourself. If Gerry did not have the foresight to look after himself, not only with me but with others, he probably would be infected. And Gerry is not emotionally or physically the strongest person in the world. And if he can say no, anybody can."

As further justification, Carl employed other metaphors as well—from finance to dance. He had insisted on this stance when explaining his own decision not to disclose to men with whom he had unprotected sex. The risks they took were not his "business." Within such contractual relationships, he had no moral responsibility.

> I went through a brief thing with an ex-friend of mine who's going toward 50, and he came to visit me and we did have unsafe sex, and several months later he said, "It's all your fault because you could have infected me," and blah blah blah, "and you knew this." And I said, "I didn't rape you. You're older than me. You know the risks as much as I do. The risks to me, what I do with myself is my business. What you do with yourself is yours." I think it takes two to tango, simple as that.

The uncertainty that swirled around definitions of "safer sex" highlighted the need for partners to protect themselves, based on their own assessments. As an uninfected gay man, Oscar took the message of self-protection seriously. "What I consider protection is not what somebody else would consider protection. Generally I think it's very important for people to really say that each person is responsible for his own health." Ben weighed the "murky" risks and benefits and concluded that individuals were making their own assessments and that therefore he was not responsible for making these judgments for others.

Still, how far could this disavowal of responsibility toward others extend? Even some who adopted a position of caveat emptor would, when pressed, draw limits on a "seller's" freedom. Morris, the uninfected gay man, saw the failure to protect oneself as a foolish refusal to deal with the ever-present dangers of sex. Nevertheless, he drew a dramatic moral distinction between silence and lies. His experience was defined by his relationship with an infected lover. "I feel that it's the responsibility of both partners, and I think probably everybody these days needs to assume that everybody's positive and needs to function under that assumption. If they don't, I think that's probably their own denial. I think a lot of times people don't want to know." But he saw deception in sexual encounters as morally unacceptable. "I think if you're lying, if someone is operating on information that you've given them and you have a trust and you've actually lied to them, then I think that that's pretty reprehensible. I believe in someone's word, and I think that actively deceiving somebody is not right."

Holding Partners to Account

Others vigorously rejected comparisons between the ethics of sexual intimacy and those of the commercial encounter, where moral norms existed, even if minimally constraining. While urging individuals to protect themselves, they held those who transmitted HIV morally accountable.

Some drew clear moral lines. Oliver, the uninfected Louisianan, had organized a sex club for uncircumcised gay men. He said, "The buyer should always beware, but also the seller should be punished when he's selling inferior goods, if you or someone knows about it and can prove it. I think to spread this around is about the worst thing you can do in today's society at all."

At the heart of this outlook was the role of intention. As Tony, the bisexual former injecting-drug user, said, "It's one thing to sin, but to know you are sinning is worse." Ernest, the screenwriter, wouldn't have blamed himself if he had infected someone, because it wouldn't have been done intentionally. "It's like a dumb mistake, but an honest mistake." A willful act that placed someone at risk, however, engendered moral responsibility. With the specter of HIV transmission informing his words, Marvin, the postal worker, spoke about a woman he knew.

> I met a young lady who worked in the telephone company who had a boyfriend who gave her the clap. He knew he had the clap, but didn't tell her. Her clap proceeded to the point where, when I had to take her to her doctor, she could hardly get in my car. Once she went to the doctor and got it treated, what she learned after she got back with that same boyfriend was that it destroyed her ability to reproduce. So the sadness of it was she was very angry that her boyfriend knew he had a venereal disease, but all he wanted to do was get off and not be bothered with telling her. And this is something I've

seen happen many times over in my community circle, the men being macho in their thinking—"I don't even tell the bitch, you know, all I want to do is get off." And it's an attitude about self, an attitude about responsibility to the individual that you're with.

Even when condoms were used, some believed that, given the gravity of the associated risks, nondisclosure about HIV represented a moral failure. *Safer* sex was not *safe* sex, and any risk required that the unsuspecting partner be given the opportunity to choose in the light of full disclosure. Tom, the uninfected former priest, celibate until his late thirties, said,

> I think it's wrong to endanger somebody. I think for me to have somebody get in my car if I know the brakes are bad, and say we're going to go on an hour and a half trip together, I think I've got to tell them there's a little bit of risk. I think just to say I've got a condom on is not enough. I just think you can't withhold information when you have the information and when you're putting the person at any risk. Nobody can tell me and expect me to believe that somebody isn't uncomfortable the next day or a week or two later when they find out that the person they were with does have HIV. They immediately think back, now what did we do? And they squirm a little bit when they think of the deep kissing. They squirm a bit with the oral sex. They don't say, oh, those are in the minimal risk categories. There's a bit of resentment or anger. I think that's a loaded gun and unpardonable. I would consider that as dangerous as if somebody knows that they have TB and they don't take the precautions. They're just totally irresponsible, totally. I know this is very harsh and judgmental language, but you just have to draw certain lines.

For Tom, safer sex—with its risks, however small—did not preclude the need for full disclosure.

In these judgments, the image of the dangerous weapon repeatedly arose. Sam, the infected respiratory therapist, also compared HIV to "a loaded gun" and said that individuals had responsibility not just for themselves but for their partners. "It takes two to tango, yes, and it's like if you have a loaded gun and you're going around pointing it. So you should tell them before. Then, if they choose to accept it, that's a different story. Even then I don't even know if that would be acceptable to me." Comparisons to drunk driving emerged as well. Ernest, who believed he had been infected by a former girlfriend who didn't know she was infected, said, "It seems like a basic precept that you shouldn't kill somebody, you shouldn't get in a car drunk and drive at seventy miles an hour, or drive at all, or operate heavy machinery. It's protecting other people from your own acts."

Ongoing relationships in particular were thought to require disclosure based on basic principles of trust, decency, and respect. Nancy, infected by a lover who had injected drugs, voiced this position firmly. "If they know, they have to tell because he's consciously infecting her, maybe killing her, and that's not right. He definitely has the obligation. If he has any humanity in him, or any love toward this other person, he's got to tell her. You can't go around tattooing people, but I think it's something that you have to tell."

Those who condemned such behavior often viewed it, as did Claudio, as "a fucked-up crime." Lance, the recovering alcoholic, shared this view, although as recently as two years earlier he had engaged in unsafe sex without disclosure with strangers. "You're committing a crime. It's sort of like attempted murder, and that's not right. I don't care, confidential or not, no one has that right. The other party has the right to be apprised of your physical condition."

Women especially vilified men who placed their female partners at risk. Wilma, the homeless woman who learned of her infection when her son was diagnosed with AIDS, saw men who failed to practice safe sex as inhuman. "They just doing it like it ain't nothing wrong. They're picking condoms out of the basket at the clinic and not using them. They're dogs. They should lock them up." Charlene, who still used drugs, was harsh as well, given that children might become infected.

> I hate to lump them all together and say they don't have a conscience, but a lot of the men I know don't. This guy . . . had the virus and was telling me the other day that this girl called him and she's six months pregnant. And now she's having a baby. I don't know if she has the virus. But how could you do that? Have you thought about if the baby is born with the virus, what you're subjecting this baby to? It's because he didn't have a conscience, he didn't care.

Nondisclosure in conjunction with unsafe sex was seen as an ultimate transgression, as evil. Punishment was due. The news of her infection stunned Jane, the middle-class woman who had had no reason to suspect a former partner was infected.

> It's just outrageous that men think it's okay not to wear condoms; that a woman can ask her partner to wear a condom and he can say, "No, I don't want to," and pressure her into having sex anyway. It's mind-boggling. I think it's evil to do that. I think it's a crime. If battering a woman is a crime, this is an even worse crime. I mean, I think it's attempted murder, and I think they should be tried and convicted.

While some could come to their ultimate judgment only after considerable inner conflict, others quickly and unambiguously viewed the issues in this way.

Many thought unprotected sex without disclosure was a moral, if not legal, crime. The views of Otis, the uninfected gay social worker, were all the more impressive given that his professional social work training might have rendered such judgments difficult.

> A lover to me is very serious: you're going to share with that person probably a little bit more than you might with your regular friends. You're sleeping together, living together. If you haven't got to a point where you can tell him your HIV status, there's something seriously missing. One partner may ask at some point, "Hey, by the way, Jim, are you positive or negative?" And the person's going to say, "Ah, no." I think that's a serious crime, maybe not in a legal sense, but it's a crime to the other person. I think it's wrong morally. Maybe that's my Catholic upbringing.

Even if the virus was not transmitted, the individual who had knowingly endangered others was morally culpable. Otis recalled an awful event on the Long Island Rail Road when a gunman opened fire on rush-hour passengers.

> Morality transcends the actuality. The guy on the Long Island Rail Road, if he never actually shot any of those people, but had every intention to but was somehow stopped beforehand, and was by all indications going to kill more people—what's the moral issue? Certainly, of course, people are dead and the actual murder can be perceived of as a most grave matter. But even if he never actually pulled the trigger but meant to, I think there's something ultimately very serious about the whole thing. Forget about the legal system. I believe in a moral system. I don't even know how I believe in it, whether it be a karma thing or some traditional religious thing. But I think no one gets off the hook.

The strongest condemnation of those who failed to inform their sexual partners of their HIV infection typically invoked religious images—used even by those who no longer identified themselves as believers. Some saw the ultimate judgment as coming from God himself. Appalled by a female friend's behavior, Beatrice, the uninfected woman who had traded sex for drugs, rejected the assertion that fear justified not informing a sexual partner. A friend had told her, "'He would beat me up. My God, he would have killed me.'" Beatrice asserted in response that "God's judgment" would, in the end, hold her to account.

> You're playing with people's lives in your hand. You have this virus, and we

are all going to have to meet our Maker. How are you going to stand up in front of God, and he knows that you had this and you did it. Come on, don't be like that. My friend said, "What you want me to do, stop having sex?" I say, "No, at least tell them before you even get ready to do something."

Others invoked more extreme religious imagery—hell itself. Maurice, infected by a lover who claimed he was surely uninfected, said about partners who don't disclose and then infect others, "I think that they're probably going to roast in hell, because when they die they're going to be dying in a state of guilt, and I think that's what hell is." Of note, Maurice had himself withheld the fact of his infection from a male sexual partner. The contrast between his firm beliefs and his own behavior illustrates how it is one thing to give voice to moral ideals, another to act on them.

Though most of those with whom we spoke agreed that disclosure or safer sex was imperative, many who held such beliefs acknowledged that they had occasionally strayed from the ideal, and they offered a variety of explanations. For example, the combination of stigma and sexual desire could breed mendacity. Ali, the former drug user who had known of his infection for five years, noted,

I always feel honesty is the best policy. But then again, I'm not always being honest. I think that everybody that is HIV should practice safe sex and tell their sexual partners. I know I don't do it because it's very hard for me to say that. It's like, hey, I got cancer, I'm gonna die. It's very hard to come to terms with that. It's something that I guess I got to work on. I won't be totally honest with the women I am with. Because I want to have sex. A lot of times people just say things to get what they want. And I think the majority of people use that tactic.

Others were embarrassed even as they sought to justify their failure to follow their own moral ideals. Tony acknowledged the discrepancy between his behavior and the moral principles he espoused. "I just think that you should tell. You should let someone else decide what risk they want to take. I couldn't enjoy being with someone if I knew I had this huge secret." Yet, although he had had sex with men since he was diagnosed, he observed,

Here's the interesting thing about that: that I don't tell men. But first of all, no one really touches me in such a way that it would be a danger to them. I don't fuck anybody, they don't really suck me. Mostly, I am the bottom. The way I've seen it is it's the gay world, and if you're gay and having sex with strangers, you'd just better assume—and I think most gay men when they meet someone new do kind of just assume—that they're positive and act accordingly. Whereas straight people still don't do that at all. The acts are different.

Nevertheless, in viewing the gulf between what he thought right and how he acted, he said, "I'm so embarrassed. It seems like everything I've said was bullshit."

It is not unusual for individuals to voice principles about how people should behave while themselves acting quite differently. Such discrepancies, if stark, prompt accusations of hypocrisy. More often we accord considerable latitude to such failings. In ordinary language, it is a mark of moral generosity to respond to such lapses by asserting, "We're only human. We're not angels." More formally, some adopt the stance of, "Judge not, lest you be judged." Indeed, to insist on moral rectitude is commonly seen as an indication of rigidity. Yet strikingly in the context of HIV, where life itself could be endangered, some men and women insisted on standards for others while excusing their own lapses. What can account for such discordance? By way of explanation some have asserted that "a stiff cock has no conscience." From a biological perspective, commentators have claimed that one's sexual drive emerges from the limbic system—the primitive, reptilian part of the brain—while moral behavior emerges from the higher cortex. The latter has limited albeit crucial control over the former. Less scientifically, artists have long charted the many dark chasms within the heart.

In analyzing how people framed their social conceptions of what partners owed each other, we have noted the array of metaphors and images invoked, from the exculpatory to the condemnatory, and attempts to distinguish among sexual partners based on the depths and expectations of the relationship. Moral principles played very different roles in different social settings—the same individual could be firm about the necessity of disclosure in some intimate contexts but not in others. Women and men also struggled to understand their own role in placing themselves at risk—whether as a result of weakness, desire, or misplaced trust.

Acting on Judgments

Those who judged others' behavior—such as failure to either disclose or use condoms—as unacceptable then had to decide how to respond. Should they try to persuade those placing others at risk to change this behavior? And if so, how forceful should such persuasion be? Even more difficult, was it appropriate to protect the privacy of friends who place others at risk? In the fluid dynamics of everyday life and friendships, what is the role of confidentiality? What are the ordinary rules governing the privacy of communication among friends, neighbors, and acquaintances, and how do these rules shift in the presence of a lethal threat like AIDS?

Even those who judged certain behaviors as reprehensible did not always choose to confront acquaintances who potentially endangered others. The ethos of HIV support groups—where one often hears of individuals practicing unsafe sex without disclosure—could preclude such confrontations and hence conflict with public health priorities of saving others' lives. Jane, who thought she was infected by a former lover, felt strongly that one should not place others at risk. Nevertheless, she remarked, "It's the nature of the support group. You can offer your ideas and suggestions and maybe some gentle sort of encouragement to do what you think is right. But critical confrontation is not really what the support group is about." Thus she held back, though appalled, by the behavior of an infected woman in her group who was sexually involved with an uninfected man. "When she comes to the group I don't say to her, 'I think that's outrageous that you're doing this.' But that's what I think."

More commonly, those who believed someone was behaving reprehensibly found a way to convey their views. Ali—who had acknowledged his own lapses of honesty with partners but viewed the universe as a moral place in which good and bad behaviors were rewarded or punished accordingly—used his support group to address this issue.

> There was one guy that was a dog. He would have unsafe sex with HIV. And I thought, man, what are you doing? But he was so proud of just getting women. I had a confrontation with him, but I had to back away because I would have come to his level, and I don't need stress in my life. He was just talking about some crazy shit that he was going through, and it sounded like BS to me, and I confronted him on it, and he jumped up—and you don't do that in the group, you just talk about what you're going through, you don't threaten anybody physically. I sat there and smiled, because I wasn't going to let that get me, but after the meeting was over I pulled him aside. I said, "You know what I have for you, man, is that you're sitting there talking about what you did to this woman, and all the time you probably could have hurt her. Down the pipeline," I said, "what goes around comes around, remember that."

Attempts to change behavior could be made not only in such group contexts but among friends and acquaintances—sometimes with considerable thought as to what might be most effective. Marvin, the uninfected postal worker who once contracted syphilis, was sufficiently concerned about a friend's behavior to warn him, but to little avail.

> I spent a great deal of time with a friend who is HIV positive. His habit would
> be to go out on a Friday night, get some cocaine or something like that, play
> around at the piers, suck cock, things of that nature, and he'd come to spend
> time with me early on a Saturday or Sunday morning to wind down from his
> drug binge and to catch sleep before he went home to his more wealthy envi-
> ronment and be able to present himself with composure to his father, so he
> wouldn't look like a cat that was dragged out of the street. He'd say, "Boy I
> met this one or that one, etc.," and I'd say to him, "Well did you tell that per-
> son that you were HIV positive?" "No, I didn't think I needed to, because . . ."
> So a lot of our conversations would hinge around this subject matter, and it
> troubled me a great deal because on many occasions he would not tell them.
> Oftentimes he felt bad in talking to me, because he felt like I was putting a
> damper on his activities. It gave him too much consciousness of his responsi-
> bility to his partner.

When efforts to change others' dangerous behavior failed, it was necessary to consider whether one had a right or duty to warn those who were
endangered. Confidentiality was seen as paramount. Patrick, the police officer who masked his bisexuality and had wrestled with how to disclose to his
fiancée, thought that no matter how much he might have endangered
others, he would have been profoundly injured if his HIV status had been di-
vulged. It was his secret to reveal.

> If you would have told me that you were going to tell on me, I wouldn't have
> told you. I'll eventually come to grips with doing the right thing. But if some-
> one's going to tell on me, go behind me, it would be very destructive. A guy
> might have shot drugs years ago, he might have performed oral sex on every-
> thing that had two legs, and now HIV is coming on him. And I think his fear is
> of being discovered. Just to go behind somebody, like through an anonymous
> call, I think could put an incredible strain on him. I don't know how I would
> react. Maybe I'd have hurt myself or maybe just have to fucking do something,
> like, "Fuck it, I got to get out of here," rather than finally confronting it. Let the
> person confront it within themselves and as they get support and help, they
> find the world still holds up, and then they'll start to tell. It takes a while.

Given the sensitivity of the information involved, others agreed that confidentiality should be adhered to without exception. Speaking about those
who placed their sexual partners at risk, Peter, the physician closeted about
his bisexual past, said, "I think that it's wrong, not the most moral type of
behavior for someone to undertake. But at the same time, I wouldn't call up
his or her partner to say, 'You should know this about the person you're

with.' I think who someone tells is a very personal thing." Of note, he drew analogies between warning someone who was imperiled by a lover and his father's disclosing his own son's infection to a sister and her boyfriend. "I felt it wasn't his right to tell somebody else my status prior to my giving consent."

Some thought their specific role in an individual's life restricted the degree to which they could act. Keith, the former drug user, now abstinent and working for the phone company, kept warning a man he was sponsoring in AA about placing a girlfriend at risk. He felt his position as sponsor did not allow him to act further. "I don't feel like I have that kind of responsibility. I don't think I'm walking around with that kind of power to say, 'Listen: if you don't tell, I'm going to tell, because she's got to know.'"

Those who did choose to warn imperiled individuals worried about how best to issue the alarm. Many sought to do so in a way that did not directly reveal who it was that posed the danger. Ronald, a middle-aged former drug user, had a sense of responsibility that made him want to protect others.

> I said to a girl I was close to, whose man was having an affair with somebody else, "That guy, cut him loose, he's doing . . ." And she responded, "It's none of your business, why are you coming to me with that?" I don't know how it would be effective. Now what I would say would be something like, "You know, you need to be careful, there's a lot going on today," and I would share with her about sleeping with whoever it is, you're sleeping with everyone that person has ever had; and there's new viruses, all of a sudden they're monsters. Just ask her to be cautious and then maybe give her some literature.

Others warned indirectly, for example by intimating that they had additional information they could divulge. Beatrice, who was uninfected although she had traded sex for drugs, said, "I don't like to be in nobody's business." Nevertheless, when she learned that a male friend had been sexually involved with a woman she knew to be infected, "I said, 'Well, did you use a condom? I'm not gonna say no more, just go have yourself tested.'"

Warnings might be coded in a variety of ways. David, who was uninfected and had lived monogamously with his lover for ten years, was troubled that a female neighbor was dating a man whom he had met in a gay Episcopal group and whom he knew engaged in unsafe sex.

> I called him up and said, "Have you told her that you are gay or bisexual?" He said, "No, and I'm not going to." I said, "Have you got tested?" He said, "No, and I'm not going to." I thought that was being very irresponsible. So the

> woman and I were chatting, and I told her that I knew him, and that he was quite active sexually and she should be careful. That's all I said, I didn't say anything more. I felt that was enough to say. I didn't say "bisexual."

In fact, like David, many considered the depth of their relationship with an endangered person in deciding whether to warn that person that he or she was at risk. Imperiled friends were owed more than mere acquaintances. Emanuel, the now sober social worker in an AIDS service organization, said,

> I don't think it'd be my place to really say anything, unless it was somebody that I really, really felt close with. If I was close to the person at risk it would be worth it, because of my feelings toward this person. If it were less than that, it wouldn't be worth taking the risk. The guy could really go off on me, "What, are you violating my trust, violating my confidentiality?" although it's not as if he's a patient of mine.

Morris, uninfected and living with an HIV-positive lover, drew boundaries as well. "If someone I'm close to is in danger, I might reach out and protect him. But I probably wouldn't do that to a stranger. I live in a world where I've limited my scope of responsibility as much as I can. I don't get out there and play Mother Theresa to the world."

Given the gravity of HIV transmission, others rejected distinctions between friends and acquaintances. A duty of rescue knew no such boundaries. Ernest, infected years earlier by a former girlfriend who had notified him by a letter, stated about revealing another's infection, "I'm someone who respects people's privacy a lot, and I would feel nervous about doing it. But I would feel compelled to do it because I think they're endangering this person. I think it's murder."

Finally, some believed that warning was a moral imperative but were uncertain about how such notification should take place. The job might best be left to public agencies. Jim, the computer programmer who had contacted his past female but not male partners, said,

> I believe that a mechanism should exist to inform the partner. If a person can't live up to their responsibility to their lover, that doesn't remove the need for the lover to know, and I don't know whether it's the city administration or the Catholic Church or Gay Men's Health Crisis or my responsibility. I just know that a person is in dire need to know that their health is in peril. I don't see that there's a need to protect an infected person's confidentiality to the point that another person will die. There has to be some kind of a line that says that your right to kill somebody stops here.

What responsibility do we have for the behavior of our friends or acquaintances? How do we confront those who may endanger others? What are the bounds or limits of our responsibility? How do we decide? Who, if anyone, should be warned and what should be revealed in such alarms? While some saw these issues as having simple moral clarity—the endangered had a need and a right to know—others were uncertain. They were constrained by norms of privacy and conceptions of limited obligations to friends and strangers. To Cain's ancient question, "Am I my brother's keeper?" the answer was not always clear.

The English language is filled with unflattering terms to describe those who arrogate to themselves the right to intrude in the lives of others—busybodies, snoops, tattletales. Within our culture, which views privacy as critical but imperiled, warning third parties in the absence of any legal obligation to do so does not come naturally. Strikingly, to justify reticence, those who chose not to warn borrowed the prescriptive norms of confidentiality that typically govern relationships between doctors and patients, lawyers and clients. Conversely, those who chose to warn often asserted that norms of privacy had limits—that in the face of great risk, the duty to protect took precedence.

Dangerous Acts and the Limits of Professional Confidentiality

Ordinary women and men felt torn about limiting confidentiality, but how did they understand the duties of doctors and other health care professionals who knew of infected patients placing sexual partners at risk? On the one hand, a failure to adhere strictly to norms of professional confidentiality could injure those who had revealed themselves to their caregivers. On the other hand, the maintenance of strict secrecy precluded warning those who were endangered. Attitudes ranged widely.

Those with clinical training knew of the debates that whirled two decades earlier around the landmark case *Tarasoff v. Regents of the University of California,* in which the California Supreme Court ruled that a psychotherapist should be required to protect the intended victim of a patient. "The protective privilege ends," said the court in its now famous formulation, "where the public peril begins."[1] But whether or not they knew about *Tarasoff,* many of our interviewees could grasp the moral significance of the issues at stake. Confidentiality and secrecy could protect but also, as Sissela Bok noted, endanger. How did men and women with or at risk for HIV talk about these issues?

Many believed that doctors or counselors who knew of patients putting sexual partners at risk should warn those who were vulnerable. A 50-year-old woman, infected through injecting-drug use, noted about the claims of the imperiled,

> The doctor or psychiatrist should notify her and tell her. It's going to be hard for him to do so, breaking that type of news to her and knowing what it's going to do to the relationship. But being the doctor, and being that he has a profession in helping people, I feel that if I were the psychiatrist I would go and inform her and let her know regardless of what it might do to the relationship or what he might feel.

Those who supported breaching confidentiality thought the fatal nature of HIV infection set it apart from other infectious and sexually transmitted diseases. Jane, infected during an affair years earlier, felt that a transmissible disease, even an STD, did not provide sufficient warrant to breach confidentiality unless it were fatal. She said, "I just think that this is life and death stuff. This isn't syphilis. This is something that once you're exposed, you're never going to get rid of, until the day you die, and so I think things like confidentiality are sometimes superseded by the gravity of the condition."

In deciding that the principle of confidentiality should not be absolute, others drew on their own experience of HIV infection. Tony, who was infected and used condoms with both men and women, though only disclosing to his female partners, had experienced the horrors of the disease. He said, "I know what I've been through, and I know what I go through now, and I don't want anyone to have to feel that way."

Informing individuals about the risk they unknowingly faced had important benefits for them, including the start of potentially life-saving treatments. Dolores, infected by a male partner, asserted, "I think they should be able to notify the partner, because if you don't get treatment, that means you die because you don't get no treatment. You could get a common cold and it could turn into pneumonia and you could die."

Some justified limitations on confidentiality by drawing analogies to other legally prescribed restraints on medical secrecy. Ernest believed that he was infected by a woman who hadn't known she was HIV positive and who later notified him by a letter. He argued, "If this guy was going to go off and infect somebody, it would be like a guy has left my office with a loaded gun, and I know he's going to go home and start shooting in the apartment. We're not sure he's going to hit his wife. But I know he's going to go shoot in the apartment. For the doctor to go, 'Well, you know, it's not really my business,' to me, is like battered women." Tom, the former priest, said, "I think it's as dangerous as one of those child abuse type things, you have to get somebody out of the danger."

Still others, misinformed about the extent to which the law did in fact permit physicians to breach confidentiality, thought the legal system did not go far enough and unreasonably privileged privacy over the rights of the vulnerable. Fred, the infected bisexual who had told no one but his wife, parents, and physician, noted,

> If you can save that person's life from getting HIV, the doctor is morally obligated to tell that person, even if he's destroying the relationship with his patient. But you can't have that in this country. They claim everyone will clam up; no one will talk to doctors. But I don't believe that. Would I be willing to risk my livelihood and the life and financial well-being of my family to protect someone like that? I'm glad I don't ever have to make that judgment call.

Those who believed that clinicians should protect the vulnerable recognized the great logistical and moral dilemmas involved. Many believed that professionals should provide a period of time in which infected individuals could inform partners themselves. But the psychological difficulties of disclosure did not license endless prevarication. Time was not neutral when someone was being exposed to HIV. Janet, the former prostitute, was not infected, though her partner was. She noted, "Give the patient a chance, because they're scared, and they want to feel their partner out properly. Give the person a fifty-fifty chance, a chance to do right. I would give them a month. That's enough time. And if they can't do it, say, 'Well listen, I'm going to have to call them.'" She knew how difficult disclosure could be, because her lover had delayed telling her that he was infected. He later explained that he feared she would say, "What? Get the fuck out of here!" Andrew, the gay chef, shared her perspective. Of note, in so doing he chose to make his case by invoking the example of heterosexual marriage. "If I was a doctor, I would say, 'Now that we know you're infected and you're married, I'm going to give you a bit of time to think about this, and then at a certain point you're going to have to explain this to your wife. And if you do not explain this to your wife, I will explain it to her.' This is not a game. We're talking about life and death."

But even among those who believed that protection of the vulnerable was a moral imperative, some perceived the enormous inherent quandaries and uncertainties. Tom, the former priest, saw parallels with the dilemmas posed by the confessional seal.

> That's a real ethical dilemma. I would try to frame it like this: "Everything is confidential except if something is imminently dangerous to you or somebody else; then I would be obligated to say something." If the person was

threatening the other person with a gun, it'd certainly be enough. I would put it in that category. I think legally you probably aren't allowed to tell the status. If I could, I think I would. Of course, I say it, but would I? Would I lose my license? Would I go through all this?

Given the conflicting moral principles involved, some felt torn, unable to decide. Larry, the infected gay New Zealander, was pulled between the silence he thought the principle of confidentiality required "intellectually" and the breach that he felt was necessary emotionally. Given the seriousness of the cases involved, he thought physicians were "compelled to play God," either way—by failing to disclose or by intervening to protect.

However, others rejected the idea that doctors or counselors should break confidentiality. Some individuals were troubled by the potential consequences and felt the provider should instead work with the patient or client. Professionals were obliged to use their skill and training to facilitate the necessary disclosures. But violating confidentiality carried too high a cost. Sam, the infected gay respiratory therapist, described this quandary, focusing on the importance of preserving the clinical relationship.

> I can't condone someone knowingly infecting other people with HIV. But you have a right to confidentiality. As a mental health professional, there are certain codes that you have to abide by. It becomes a real dilemma. I could understand that telling the other person would completely break the relationship with the patient. You can only work as a team to work out solutions.

Pragmatic considerations should be foremost. Ironclad principle could not serve as a guide to action. These views resembled those articulated two decades earlier in the legal battles that surrounded the *Tarasoff* case: compelling psychiatrists to breach confidentiality to protect patients' intended victims would be counterproductive. Dangerous patients would simply keep their violent thoughts from their therapists. Emanuel, now a social worker following years of drug use, could not, based on his clinical perspective, accept disclosure without consent.

> It seems like it's the right thing to do on the one hand. But on the other hand, what if this scenario ensues: the patient says, "I don't want to see you anymore because you're violating my trust and confidentiality," and then the woman, who is also his patient, says, "How can you say that about Johnny? I love Johnny, we have great sex together and besides I hate condoms and I don't even think that he's positive like you say he is." Then you've lost two people. It would have been an ineffective intervention. At least you could have maybe helped them and worked toward getting him to disclose.

Those who opposed breaches in confidentiality typically asserted that clinicians who had made every effort to facilitate communication had no further ethical obligation. Remarkably, the infected as well as the uninfected held this outlook. Thus, Diane, the uninfected woman whose husband had lied about being infected, noted,

> I think doctors should get them both in the office and sit them both down and have a conference with them. They should be able to figure it out from there: "A doctor or a counselor is calling us in. There must have to be a reason behind it. Something is wrong. One of us is doing something that is not right." After the doctor has tried the first time, the second or third time, and the counselor has tried, that's it. You can take a horse to the water, but you can't make him drink.

While those who had supported breaches of confidentiality saw analogies between exposure of partners to HIV and threats of violence, those who opposed limitations to confidentiality saw the risks of HIV transmission as less serious than the dangers addressed by the *Tarasoff* decision. George, the psychologist, said,

> I've never been a directive therapist. I would certainly make a major issue out of it, and push this man to explore why he wasn't going to tell his wife, and what that meant, with the hope that if that were done well, he would of course want to tell her. But I have trouble with the issue of telling his wife, which is really a violation of therapeutic confidentiality and the basis for the whole relationship: that this is a space where people can talk about things and know that it will be kept in the room.

Aware of the weight of *Tarasoff* doctrine, he distinguished between the danger of HIV transmission and that of imminently threatened grave injury. "If somebody said to me 'I want to kill my wife,' then of course that would be different. I think again, legally and ethically, I'm bound to let this person know. But when it's much more in the gray zone, I would be more likely to explore rather than act on it."

Others elaborated on why HIV was in "the gray zone," minimizing the risks involved. Sherri, the physician, had been the subject of "people's gossip" and believed that as a physician she should encourage disclosure but not notify partners. "I don't think I would feel disclosing would be my duty or responsibility," she asserted. Her obligation was "more to my patient than to the larger good. I don't think that it's a given that if somebody's positive and you have unprotected sex, you're going to get it. It's just not like that. I don't believe it is like beating somebody up, because it's not 100 percent. I know so many couples where one person is positive, one is negative. It's nowhere near 100 percent."

Like Sherri, others also saw breaching confidentiality as an unjustifiable extension of professional authority. Morris, who was uninfected, raised this point, reflecting a leitmotif that ran through the claims of those who opposed violations of the clinical privilege. "I think that in the scheme of things, if you have a hundred patients that you test and find are positive, you will probably have more of them that you can control than not, and if you get a reputation for overstepping your bounds then you might turn off the next hundred that come into your office. I think there's a danger in that." Others, like Craig, the former male prostitute, invoked still more extreme images of the prying state. "It's none of the health care worker's business. He's not like the AIDS police, there is no such thing."

The notion of overreaching and of overstepping bounds was intimately linked to understandings of the nature of physician-patient trust. Thus, such overextension was often seen as simply wrong. Carl, who only "occasionally" disclosed to casual sexual partners, feeling it would "kill the mood," answered "absolutely not" to the question of whether the doctor should ever tell. "If I were in a situation like that where a doctor felt a need to tell my lover, I would report the doctor and I would drop him because, first of all, most especially in a doctor-patient relationship, if I can't trust you with a confidence, I'd never trust you with my life. There's just no question about that"—a perspective compatible with justifying his own nondisclosure practices.

Professional breaches of confidentiality raised, too, the specter of a slippery slope. Breaking confidentiality could perhaps be theoretically justified in a narrowly defined instance where one person was putting another at risk. Yet violating the principle of secrecy might produce a cascade of harms outweighing the possible good of informing one endangered person. Ginger, the former injecting-drug user who had suffered an unexpected bad review at work after disclosing her HIV status to her supervisor, said, "I've seen so many confidentiality issues in all of the years. I can see where this one thing makes sense for a psychiatrist to have the right to call the partner. But then that would fall over into God knows what."

Others detailed the loss of freedom that would be entailed and the broader social and political implications of forced disclosure. Ellen, the infected journalist, filled in the picture at which Ginger had only hinted. She believed that individuals with HIV had obligations not to endanger partners, but she utterly opposed imposing duties on doctors to disclose. "That would be like a Communist society. How can you enforce that? Once we start to say to the doctor that you have to tell, then what happens?" Finally, some confronted the prospect of physician disclosure with cataclysmic concerns about the fate of freedom. Bianca, the incest survivor, said,

> No, no, no, no, no. Breaches of confidentiality should never be permitted. It can be a very dangerous situation. When we're talking about people who have low self-esteem, unloved, going through all these problems. They don't have as much control as they want in their lives anyway. Just the humanity of it. You take away choice, you breach the Constitution of the United States. You can't do that. Not and still be free.

Whether supporting imposition of limits on confidentiality or maintenance of strict privacy, men and women who felt betrayed often drew on their personal experiences. Wilma, the infected former drug user and sex worker, believed that a physician had informed the father of her son that she had "some kind of female infection—a yeast infection or something—and he went stupid," abusing her and threatening her with abandonment. She said of such doctors, "They should mind their own business."

Thus, the question of whether a patient's confidentiality should ever be breached when he or she endangered a partner raised a series of controversial clinical, moral, medical, practical, and political issues. The questions that emerged ranged from the most personal to the most political. In what kind of civil society do we want to live? How should the boundary between the public and private be drawn? How should the state and professionals protect the distinctions? What circumstances might justify limits on the rules of privacy? Does the threat of HIV constitute such an extraordinary situation? The ideas that shaped men's and women's choices and beliefs reflected their understandings of broad ideological and moral imperatives. Even those for whom such conceptions were foreign sought to explain their choices in the light of their own inner sense of right or wrong and private moralities that reflected their family background, class, race, gender, sexual orientation, and experience.

Secrets in Public Life

The men and women in our study typically learned they were infected with HIV in settings where confidentiality, and sometimes anonymity, were promised. Nonetheless, from that moment on, they were forced to struggle with questions of how and with whom they should share their secret. The accounts in this book reveal the pain that many encountered in confronting these issues—the shame and rejection, even violence, they anticipated and experienced. These accounts also depict support and love. In all cases, disclosure was a monumental and defining issue, challenging and laying bare processes of decision making about morality, truth, secrets, and trust in everyday life.

These disclosure decisions—although HIV-infected individuals made every effort to keep them private—could not be matters of indifference to others concerned about the course of the AIDS epidemic. Inevitably, whether infected individuals tell their sexual partners has important implications for viral spread. Therefore, public health officials have continued to give attention to ways of encouraging and facilitating disclosure. They have faced, too, the issue of how to respond to those who fail to disclose and who engage in sexual or needle-sharing behaviors that can transmit HIV. These concerns have also captured the attention of the broader public, seized by the drama and tragedy of AIDS. The private decisions described here have become matters of public debate. On many occasions the controversy reflected an appreciation of the complexity of the issues at stake, but too often was animated by moral fury. Controversy has centered on two broad questions that touch on the history of public health responses to infectious disease: contact investigations and coercive control of those who threaten the public well-being.

Partner Notification

Current policy debates can best be understood in historical and political contexts. From the early 1980s, public health officials confronting the AIDS epidemic had come to recognize the crucial importance of confidentiality. Those at risk for HIV infection could be encouraged to undergo counseling and testing only if convinced that their test results would not be disclosed without their consent. Thus, the Centers for Disease Control and Prevention, the surgeon general, the Institute of Medicine, the National Academy of Sciences, and the Presidential Commission on the HIV Epidemic all stressed that the protection of confidentiality did not compromise the protection of public health.[1] On the contrary, confidentiality was a precondition for achieving public health goals.

The consensus masked underlying tensions. Public health officials, AIDS activists, gay rights organizers, and civil liberties groups supported the protection of confidentiality. However, for some, the protection of privacy was critically important but not an absolute. Others saw the demands of confidentiality as inviolate. Thus, conflict was inevitable over the development of public programs for reaching out to those who were unknowingly in danger. The controversy focused on whether, in the context of AIDS, either of two public health approaches to informing those at risk was appropriate.[2]

The first, as described in Chapter 6, involves the "duty to warn." This approach arose out of clinical settings in which physicians knew the identities of endangered persons and was a radical departure from the professional norm of confidentiality. Typically it required that imperiled individuals be warned even against the wishes of the patient and whatever the consequences for privacy.

The second approach—partner notification or contact tracing—emerged from STD-control programs in which the clinician typically did not know beforehand the identity of those who might have been exposed. This approach required patients to cooperate voluntarily in providing the names of their contacts. The index patient's identity was never disclosed to the notified party, and absolute confidentiality was guaranteed in the notification process.

Yet despite four decades of experience with contact tracing for other STDs, in the first years of the HIV epidemic, efforts to undertake such public health interventions met with fierce resistance. Activists and civil libertarians worried that contact tracing would compromise the privacy of both index patients and their former partners.[3] Furthermore, opponents argued that HIV, because of its uniquely stigmatized status, was not like other STDs.

This opposition shaped the initial response of public health officials, especially in states or cities with relatively large numbers of AIDS cases. In San Francisco, for example, a proposal that health department staff offer contact-tracing services to bisexual men whose female partners might unknowingly have been placed at risk was denounced as Orwellian, because of the prospect of health departments creating lists of bisexual men and their partners.[4] Even greater antagonism greeted the possibility of creating lists of the male contacts of gay men, because of fears of discrimination. In Minnesota, an especially bitter controversy erupted over the state's effort to launch an aggressive contact-tracing program in 1986. One opponent declared that "the road to the gas chamber began with lists in Weimar Germany."[5] The hyperbole that often characterized the dispute revealed the depths of fear in the most AIDS-affected communities. This concern could not be readily assuaged by matter-of-fact recitations about the exemplary records of health department efforts to control sexually transmitted disease. AIDS was different.

Underlying this debate was the fact that in the first years of the AIDS epidemic, no therapy could be offered to asymptomatic infected individuals. Thus, the role of contact tracing in the context of HIV infection differed radically from its role in the context of other STDs. In the latter case, effective treatments could be offered to notified partners; once treated and cured, they would no longer pose a threat of transmission. For HIV, nothing could be offered other than information about possible exposure to the virus.

Proponents of partner notification acknowledged the difference between AIDS and treatable STDs, but believed that such efforts could target prevention measures to those most at risk for transmitting or acquiring HIV. To opponents, on the other hand, the very effort to reach out to such individuals intruded on privacy, imposing burdens with little or no compensating benefit. General education, they asserted, could alter behavior more effectively and efficiently.

Although by the late 1980s all states were establishing the capacity to offer partner-notification services at the request of the index patient, less than half emphasized such an approach.[6] In part this fact was a reflection of lingering political resistance; in part it reflected assumptions about the costs and benefits of such interventions. Indeed, by the early 1990s the debate over contact tracing had largely shifted focus from ethical issues of privacy to questions of efficacy.[7] Early misapprehensions about the extent to which public health officials might rely on overt coercion, and the degree to which confidentiality might be compromised, had all but vanished. Increasingly, earlier experiences with contact tracing for STDs were recognized as successful in protecting the anonymity of index cases and the confidentiality of those who were contacted. Treatments for HIV had also improved, making the notification of asymptomatic individuals seem more urgent.

With political concerns allayed, many, but by no means all, gay leaders recognized that partner notification could be a "useful tool" in efforts to control AIDS.[8] Nevertheless, a vast gulf remained between recognition that partner notification could, in principle, play a role and actual implementation of such efforts. It is striking that none of the women and men with whom we spoke spontaneously offered objection to partner-notification programs. Indeed, some, without knowledge of the technical details, believed that public agencies should play a role in notifying the unsuspecting. A few saw the failure to do so as troubling.

In contrast, those we interviewed disagreed sharply about the duty to warn. The dispute mirrored the deep and lingering debate in the policy arena, stemming from the *Tarasoff* case (discussed in Chapter 6). To those who held doctor-patient communications sacrosanct, the *Tarasoff* decision, which imposed an affirmative duty on clinicians to warn or protect endangered third parties, was a profound mistake. The controversy surrounding *Tarasoff* shaped debates about whether it was ever appropriate to breach the confidentiality of HIV-positive patients who engaged in high-risk sex and failed to disclose to sexual or needle-sharing partners.

While AIDS activists and many of those interviewed for this book remained unalterably opposed to any breaches of confidentiality, others disagreed. As legal scholars and ethicists have confronted this issue, they have often concluded that breaches of confidentiality could, in special circumstances, be justified.[9] Many whom we interviewed shared this view that protection from danger took precedence over preservation of confidentiality. But even among those willing to acknowledge that the need for confidentiality was not absolute, disagreement continued over whether disclosures by physicians should be morally obligatory or discretionary; whether the moral obligation should be a legal duty; whether, in warning contacts, the identity of the index patient should be revealed; and, most importantly, whether, in the end, strict adherence to confidentiality would ultimately be more protective of the public health than a regime that countenanced or required breaches.

The American Psychiatric Association, despite opposing the *Tarasoff* decision, declared in 1987 that if patients refused to change their behavior or to notify at-risk partners, it was "ethically *permissible* to notify [the person] believed to be endangered."[10] The American Academy of Family Physicians went further and declared in 1990 that a physician who failed to convince an HIV-infected patient to inform at-risk sexual partners had an ethical obligation to breach confidentiality. The rights of the endangered party "superseded" the patient's right to privacy.[11] When the American Medical Association adopted a similar position, its president declared, "This is a landmark in the history of medical ethics. We are saying for the first time that, because of the danger to the public health and the danger to unknowing partners the physician may be required to violate patient confidentiality. The physician has a responsibility to inform the spouse. This is more than an option. This is a professional responsibility."[12]

These moves by the medical establishment alarmed gay rights and AIDS advocates and defenders of civil liberties. Those who had garnered support from public health officials for ironclad confidentiality protections, and had succeeded in getting such protections enacted into state law, saw these professional assertions as a dire turn of events. Faced with such dispute, many public health officials sought to chart a middle course, one that recognized the importance of both confidentiality and the notification of at-risk individuals. Instead of advocating *Tarasoff*-like mandatory notifications, these public health officials typically argued for a "privilege to disclose."[13] Doctors could use their professional judgment in deciding whether or not a breach of confidentiality was justified. But this political compromise was ultimately vulnerable to charges that granting physicians broad discretion could mean some individuals who were at risk would not in fact be notified. By 2000, both federal and state policy makers increasingly thought that physicians should be required to notify patients' sexual partners known to be at risk.[14] Indeed, New York State enacted legislation requiring physicians to inform the state health department of the names of spouses imperiled by their husbands or wives.[15]

Dangerous Acts and State Control

Inevitably, the question of how to confront infected individuals who endanger unsuspecting partners extends beyond the debate on confidentiality. Does such behavior warrant public health control and, if so, should such efforts entail counseling and persuasion or coercion? Does the criminal law have any role to play?

Those most concerned about protecting civil liberties and avoiding coercive measures have argued that criminal law and other control measures might be counterproductive to interrupting the spread of HIV, and that better, more effective education and counseling is the sole appropriate response to dangerous behavior. Education might change the behavior of those viewed as "recalcitrant" and, more important, could teach uninfected individuals how to protect themselves.[16] In the end, as we noted in the introduction to this book, the opponents of coercive measures asserted that self-protection was the ultimate defense against infection.

However, others concluded that such an approach was inadequate, that the state had a responsibility to protect the vulnerable, and that sexual partners, especially women, are not always able to protect themselves.[17] Those who asserted that strict enforcement measures were imperative often spoke with a moral fury, animated as much by hatred for gay men and drug users as by concerns for the public health. But that was not always the case. Clearly, many whom we interviewed thought it morally wrong to engage in unprotected sexual intercourse without disclosure. Some who held such views advocated legal sanctions.

A number of commentators who have sought to avoid coercion as a general rule see no alternative under extreme circumstances when the behavior is egregious. They perceive two options: using public health powers, including the authority to quarantine, or invoking criminal law sanctions.[18] During the formative years of the response to the AIDS epidemic, advocates of the use of public health powers typically recognized that much of the public health law for dealing with those who create risk, including the law of quarantine, was archaic.[19] Such an approach to public health threats—the product of an earlier period in the history of medicine—failed to protect due process or specify whether isolation or quarantine should be used only after other, less restrictive measures had been exhausted.[20] But while acknowledging the need to modernize public health law, these advocates believed that such authority could potentially make an important, albeit limited, contribution to preventing the spread of HIV infection by isolating those who persisted in behaviors linked to the spread of a lethal disease.[21]

In the first decade of the AIDS epidemic, twenty-five states enacted revised public health statutes that could restrict or quarantine individuals who engaged in behaviors that might spread disease. Yet despite such authority, public health officials rarely used these powers. Neither California nor New York, which together accounted for close to 40 percent of AIDS cases in the United States, did so.[22] Somewhat more common, but still unusual, public health officials issued warnings to individuals whose behavior might be dangerous. These interventions could mandate counseling or threaten criminal prosecution if behavior did not change.

Criminal law has been used more frequently than public health powers.[23] Whether under AIDS-specific statutes or the provisions of general criminal law, prosecutors have brought various charges—from attempted murder to assault with a dangerous or deadly weapon to reckless endangerment—

against infected individuals who exposed others to the risk of HIV. Cases arose from instances of spitting, biting, or blood spattering by infected individuals—actions that posed virtually no risk—but most commonly from unprotected sexual activity. Such prosecutions all too commonly failed to distinguish between patently dangerous acts and acts involving more remote or theoretical risks.

Those who believe criminal law can act as a deterrent have defended criminalization of HIV transmission. They also have invoked the retributive role of the criminal law: some acts, they hold, are so egregious and so violate the norms of decency that they deserve to be punished. Willful or negligent exposure of a partner to HIV without disclosure deserves punishment, they argue, even while acknowledging that the potential deterrent effects of such criminal sanctions are very limited.[24]

Opponents of criminal sanctions typically have pointed out the absence of evidence for the public health benefits of such laws. Moreover, they argue that threats of punishment are counterproductive and "drive the epidemic underground" by discouraging at-risk individuals from learning their HIV status. Finally, they view the punitive thrust of the criminal law as regressively harsh when applied to men and women with a fatal infection—unworthy of a society that sees itself as guided by norms of compassion.[25]

In 1998 the governor of Alaska and the state epidemiologist voiced this perspective in a message vetoing a statute to criminalize HIV transmission: "HIV is a public health problem, not a criminal problem . . . Building a trusting cooperative environment is the lynch-pin of public health success, without which numerous diseases such as tuberculosis, syphilis, and diphtheria would not have been brought under control . . . Punishing individuals will not prevent disease transmission, and providing criminal sanctions against HIV will not make it safe for uninfected individuals to engage in unsafe behaviors."[26] While expressing "outrage" against individuals who demonstrated gross indifference to the well-being of others, the governor expressed concern that the proposed statute would only further stigmatize people with AIDS.

Some who at first generally opposed the application of criminal law to the AIDS epidemic and stressed how punishment is a desperate grasping for a "fool's gold"—costly, time consuming, and ultimately of little public health significance—have come to acknowledge a very limited role for such sanctions. By acknowledging that, in especially egregious cases, criminal law has a role, they sought to defang the movement to extend the scope of punitive responses to HIV transmission.

Wisdom would dictate that these legal decisions attend to the experiences of those whose lives have been indelibly marked by the AIDS epidemic and consider the ways in which the law would affect the transmission of HIV. Ultimately, it is against that yardstick and its implication for the saving of lives that policy must be judged.

Despite controversies over the ethics and efficacy of the criminal law for almost two decades, statutes punishing at least some acts involving the threat of HIV transmission have spread. By the end of the 1990s, twenty-seven states had enacted specific statutes making HIV transmission a felony offense.[27] Four additional states classed such acts as misdemeanors. However, despite the intensity of debate on this matter, over the course of the epidemic fewer than four hundred prosecutions for HIV transmission–related acts have been recorded nationwide. The debate remains far from settled, and in coming years further legislation and court decisions will surely attempt to tackle these issues.

Between the Public and the Private

We began our inquiry by exploring morally freighted terms such as *secrets, lies, concealment,* and *trust.* In listening to women and men infected with HIV or living in the shadow of risk, in traveling through the world of what some have called "HIV land,"[28] we have gained a deeper appreciation of the complexities of truth telling in everyday life. And we have come to understand how hard it is to wrestle with the issues involved, how difficult it is to communicate about what Erving Goffman called "spoiled identity,"[29] even when people want to and feel they should.

As seen in the narratives presented in this book, the path from learning about being infected and its attendant secrets to self-revelation or going public can be long and complex. Like the process of accepting death and dying, powerfully illuminated by Elisabeth Kübler-Ross, coming to grips with a diagnosis as serious as HIV entails a range of emotions—denial, depression, anger, and acceptance. Responses are not necessarily discrete and consecutive. A host of political, social, interpersonal, and intrapsychic factors influence the process of accepting and then disclosing one's HIV infection. Disclosure is affected by, and in turn affects, these emotional states.

As we learned from these interviews, truth and lies are communicated in specific temporal, spatial, and social contexts. We were impressed by how arduous it could be to lead up to the moment of disclosure. There were problems in raising new and unwelcome subjects that shifted the mood. How was one to raise the topic in the course of a relationship or an evening? It is one thing to acknowledge the imperative "thou shalt disclose," quite another to figure out how to do it. All of this could take time. But from a moral viewpoint, when transmission is a risk, time takes on profound signif-icance. Delay, however understood, can have fatal implications.

Again and again through these accounts, we have been struck by the diffi-culty of choices faced under the shadows of uncertainty. The uninfected had to make troubling assessments of whether to believe what they were told by their sexual partners. Infected people might communicate in ambig-uous ways through codes, cues, and clues that were difficult to interpret. For many of these men and women, trust in relationships was inherent, vis-ceral—not based on cognitive assessments of risks. Trust was a de facto part of entering a committed relationship—in fact, part of the definition of com-mitment itself. Yet to act on trust might expose the uninfected to a lethal vi-rus. On the other hand, to choose not to accept the word of a partner could impair the development of a relationship. Even when uninfected individ-uals decided to protect themselves until establishing a foundation of trust, agonizing questions remained about when that moment had arrived. Some felt it never came. Almost all wrestled with the dilemma that social life re-quired some degree of trust—the faith that those we let into our lives won't hurt us—despite the lingering possibility of danger.

Infected men and women, too, had to act in the face of ambiguity, choos-ing between the benefits of concealment—of "passing"—and those of dis-closure. They had to weigh the need to share their secret with family memb-ers and friends who might provide love and support against the risk of being burdensome and being rejected or betrayed. They sought guides but found little certainty. Decisions about whether to disclose to sexual partners posed the most difficult questions. Disclosure could lead to painful rejection and end relationships that provided not only erotic pleasure but economic and emotional security as well. But failing to tell the truth could be a deception, a betrayal of trust that could kill, depending on the riskiness of the sexual behavior.

No one we interviewed had explicitly sought to spread HIV, although some women told of men whose disregard for the consequences of their acts suggested culpability. More commonly, those who did not reveal their infec-tions and engaged in behaviors that could transmit HIV did so in contexts such as baths, sex clubs, or commercial sex encounters, where they could take refuge in the thought that partners would recognize the presence of risk. But in the context of loving relationships, those who did not disclose were painfully aware of the danger of their behavior. They struggled with themselves, aware of the conflict between their acts and their moral under-standings. Fear, shame, and dread of abandonment haunted them. They ra-tionalized their behavior or lived with intense and biting guilt. Yet guilt was often not enough. A degree of guilt prodded some to disclose, while others bore these feelings for extended periods rather than divulge.

As we listened to these women and men, the moral issues of truth telling, concealment, and deception were clarified but not made simpler. Lies, we had thought, would be rather simple to identify and judge. After all, proscriptions against mendacity are enmeshed in the social fabric. Few criticisms damn as much as calling someone a liar. Perhaps as a result, when we are caught in a lie, and even when we admit our guilt, we must offer explanations or justifications. Nevertheless, we all lie. Empirical studies suggest how ubiquitous lying is—one effort to quantify suggests that college students admit to lying about twice a day.[30]

The reprehensibility of a lie depends very much on its consequences. Lies that injure differ from those that seek to protect. Repeatedly, the men and women with whom we spoke underscored this point. In addition, we found that the very definition of what constituted a lie differed. In some families, for example, the demand for openness was so powerful that not telling at all and telling lies—sins of omission and commission—were viewed as equivalent. Nevertheless, individuals generally appreciated that lying to protect children and elderly parents might be sad but was not a moral breach. The men and women we interviewed also condoned lying to those who had no right to know—employers, insurance companies, landlords, or prying neighbors.

When it came to lovers, sexual partners, and spouses, the moral issues became starker. Some viewed lying about one's HIV infection to such individuals as morally tainted, even "evil"—using terms reserved for the most extreme moral condemnation. Many could understand why, at least initially, it might be necessary to communicate indirectly. Codes could spare someone from having to mouth such painful words as "I have AIDS" or "I have HIV." But clearly, deceptive or indecipherable codes were a form of dissembling.

Keeping secrets, as we have seen, could be viewed as a form of lying or a justifiable act of self-protection, but was understood to serve other functions as well. Secrets could isolate but create group cohesiveness, too. Indeed, in "secret societies," from Masonic lodges to fraternities, the act of keeping a secret matters more than the content of the secret itself. Secretiveness functions as a way of distinguishing between us and them, one's own social group and others, as a way of providing a social glue. For women and men with HIV, the secretiveness afforded by the confidentiality in almost all clinical settings facilitated their entry into treatment. In organizations composed of people with HIV, secrecy could provide the social space for sought-after support. Sadly, though, the shame of HIV is such that some remained secretive even with other infected individuals or those who could offer emotional succor.

Our interviews also revealed the importance of understanding the secret kept from oneself in self-deception. As they spoke about themselves and others, many men and women acknowledged how they had tried to minimize the extent to which they were, in fact, at risk for HIV. They spoke of "being in denial," a term used by mental health professionals to describe defenses against threatening realities. But while therapists define this defense as unconscious, those we interviewed used the term far more loosely and broadly, suggesting at times merely a low level of awareness. Hence, while these men and women might see "denial" that existed beyond consciousness as understandable and exculpating, on other occasions they viewed self-deception as inexcusable, especially when it led to transmission of HIV to a sexual partner. How, then, was self-deception to be assessed? Could unconsciously "chosen" denials be subject to moral judgment?

The narratives presented here limn the complex range of moral norms, rules, and beliefs that govern the intimacies of everyday life. People from different educational and religious backgrounds, many of whom had not completed high school, examined with sophistication troubling moral issues about the nature of trust and ethics. Regardless of the complexity or the simplicity of the language used, ethical concerns ran wide and deep. Many articulated a view of a universe in which injurious actions were punished: do not harm others, "what goes around comes around," and the Golden Rule. Some spoke of a need to judge, others resisted such assessments, in both cases offering moral arguments to support their position. Most striking was how these women and men groped to find ways to understand and describe these issues.

The complexities provided by this range of accounts offer a context for revisiting the critical moral issues raised in our introduction by the work of Sissela Bok and David Nyberg. Like Bok, we believe the ability to preserve intimate secrets is central to the ability to shape one's life. The accounts presented here underscore this point in forceful ways. With friends, families, and co-workers, such decisions may be the cause of hurt, even bitter disappointment. As infected men and women so poignantly revealed, silence, when the risks of disclosure seem to outweigh the benefits, carried its own burden. To observers it might seem right, even best, for individuals with HIV to shed their secrets, come out, lift the weight of hiding, with its inevitable dissimulations. Thus, the failure to reveal one's HIV infection may seem foolish, sad, regrettable, even reprehensible. In the end, however, decisions about when, what, and to whom to disclose must remain with those who bear the secret. No moral calculus could justify intrusions on that right of self-determination or would be compatible with an essential respect for human dignity. Further, as we have seen, prying efforts to dislodge secrets may create the very circumstances under which people believe they have no alternative but to lie.

However, is there not only a right but a duty to remain secretive in certain circumstances? David Nyberg poses this question in warning about the hazards of truth dumping that might cause pain. Here, too, our interviews provided insights into the everyday moral universe of men and women facing the reality or prospects of terrible disease. Most remarkably, not a single individual asserted that telling the whole truth to someone who might suffer as a consequence was appropriate. Indeed, we were struck by how concern for children and elderly parents informed choices even by women and men whose history of drug use and criminal behavior might suggest disregard for others' interests and needs. At considerable cost, silence seemed morally right. Thus, Bok's strictures against protective lying veer wide of the mark, and Nyberg's observation that we owe each other more than the truth seems apt.

Yet in turning to the question of truth telling between sexual intimates, the story changes. Here, Bok and Nyberg concur: secrets, lies, dissimulations that endanger others are reprehensible. Almost always, those we interviewed agreed that they owed the truth to long-term partners, even when sexual practices posed small or remote risks. However, our respondents disagreed about whether they had a duty to reveal to casual or anonymous partners and whether low- or no-risk sexual practices vitiated such an obligation, to the extent that it existed. Some we interviewed adopted a convenient and easy moral stance—if not asked, they would not tell. In the face of danger, they embraced an ethics that permitted partners to assume risk willingly. Individuals who voluntarily entered relationships where hazards should be assumed could not blame partners who dissimulated or remained silent about being infected. But is such a stance morally acceptable? Are partners who don't ask responsible for not knowing? Inevitably, perceptions of and tolerances for risk have an impact on such assessments. How should the level of risk affect our judgments? Does the moral calculus change when a risk is only 2 percent as opposed to 20 percent? To some, 2 percent may seem minimal. Others may believe that when life is at stake, *any* risk is intolerable. In consensual relationships, who should define the acceptable?

These intimate choices pose critical questions for public morality and the ethics of a public health that seeks to enhance community well-being. That people may willingly or knowingly place themselves at risk does not end the discussion but simply raises additional questions of how such decisions should be judged and, if such choices are deemed unacceptable, what public health responses are appropriate. Society has, for example, prohibited dueling, a consensual activity, but it recognizes that heterosexual couples in which one person is infected may take grave risks to have children. Where in this spectrum does mutual risk taking by sexual partners with potentially fatal consequences fall? When such shared risk taking occurs, does "informed consent" preclude moral judgment? Does a willingness to assume risk make one morally free to impose risk?

In law and ethics, intent matters. And it is critical, too, in the moral experiences of everyday life. When someone says "I'm sorry," "it was an accident" or an "honest mistake," or merely "oops," we respond accordingly; we judge differently those who injure willfully and those who injure through negligence. On the other hand, we judge harshly those responsible for serious harms that could reasonably have been foreseen or that result from a reckless disregard for norms of safety.

For public health, none of this matters very much. What counts is transmission, whatever the motives of those who impose or take risk. And from this perspective, the morally most egregious acts may be of far less significance than the morally most ambiguous. In fact, given what we know from both epidemiology and the fine-grained accounts in this volume, HIV continues to spread not from malevolence but from sexual behaviors and drug use that do not entail a wish to harm others.

Thus, the public health challenge is to shape policies that will affect the collective behavior of those who have HIV or are at risk. Here, an appreciation of both the psychological and the moral wellsprings of intimate choices is crucial. How can health care providers and policy makers motivate HIV-infected individuals to understand the moral and social significance of decisions to reveal, hide, or lie? What role should community-based groups and public health departments play in fostering such awareness? Is it possible to characterize some behavior as morally troubling, even deplorable, without opening the way to state interventions? Is the failure to invoke the authority of the state in such circumstances morally problematic?

Since the early 1980s, such intensely personal considerations, as described here, have set the stage for policies intended to confront the AIDS epidemic. In addressing these matters, policy makers have drawn on their own ideologies on the importance of privacy, public health and safety, and the role of coercive measures in fighting epidemics. But they have also had to rely on their own understandings of the worlds of people with or at risk of HIV infection. Some who sought to formulate policy have acted in the face of total ignorance. Others have sensitively balanced the needs of public health with the fears and needs of people infected with or at risk of HIV. When policy makers have been insensitive to the fears, concerns, and needs of infected men and women, the result has been neglect or punitive actions that fail to protect the public health. In general, AIDS policy in the United States has avoided the pitfalls of a mindless embrace of coercion, in large part through the extraordinary efforts of activists—many of whom were infected—and their allies, inside and outside government.

The world of policy makers contrasts sharply with that of individuals infected with HIV. The latter struggle daily with burdens of illness and dilemmas of whether and how to tell others about their medical condition. Policy makers operate in a public realm; individuals with HIV in a private, intimate, often secretive one. The policy makers' realm is filled with abstract "populations." Individuals with HIV live in a world of husbands, wives, lovers, sexual partners, friends, and family members who may expect information—resulting in shifting and tangled interpersonal dynamics.

To be effective in limiting the spread of HIV infection and encouraging disclosure and protective sexual behavior, public efforts will need to appreciate the diversity of lives and cultures affected by the epidemic. The norms and expectations of heterosexual marriage contrast markedly with those of courtship and dating. The mores and expectations within gay communities differ even more dramatically. Thus, while the goals of public health policy may be singular—preventing the spread of HIV—intervention strategies may require exquisite sensitivity and flexibility. But sensitivity and flexibility do not mean uncritical acceptance. Occasionally, the culture or communal norms that shape individual behavior will need to be changed. For example, culturally sanctioned notions of male dominance place women at special risk for HIV.

Within this broad challenge to public health, the law can play important roles. It can foster openness and disclosure by proscribing discriminatory practices that make secrecy seem the only reasonable course. It can assure access to needed care. It can also draw a sharp line reflecting a broad social consensus as to which behaviors represent utterly unacceptable threats. But ultimately, in many ways, the role of law is very limited. How could it be otherwise, when sexual partners communicate intimately with each other, where ambiguity is often the norm, and where definitions, even of basic terms such as *disclosure, truth, lies, risk,* and *safer sex,* provoke disagreement? Moreover, law can do little to inform the difficult choices that men and women face in everyday life, in deciding about telling parents, children, friends, and colleagues.

Precisely because of a recognition of the limitations of the law, since the epidemic's earliest days, education has been viewed as the pillar of AIDS prevention. Yet this approach has had mixed results. Efforts at education have been hobbled by cultural and religious forces seeking to impose moralistic constraints on what can be said to children, adolescents, and gay men. As we have noted, even those committed to uncensored education have also debated how best to shape interventions. How should sexual partners balance the important lessons of self-protection—always use condoms—against those that dictate an obligation to disclose? Can an educational campaign simultaneously encourage both skepticism and trust?

Education and counseling rely on nurses, doctors, and other health care professionals, but do not always occur. The increasing proportion of people with HIV who have entered clinical care has furthered a dependence on clinicians. But at the end of the 1990s, five years after the introduction of powerful antiretroviral therapies, the available evidence has been disappointing. One study, for example, found that one-third of patients had not been counseled about safer sex by providers, and half had never been spoken to about disclosure. At this most basic level, then, public health messages were not reaching the HIV-infected.[31]

In addition to the focus on education and counseling, by the late 1980s a consensus emerged that safeguarding people with HIV against discrimination would substantially protect the nation's health and counter the stigma that prompted fears of disclosure. But stigmatization continued, an expression of cultural forces resistant to change—latent and manifest homophobia, racism, and fear of and revulsion toward injecting-drug use. As a consequence, despite the gradually increasing visibility of HIV and the social acceptance of people with AIDS, numerous infected individuals still feel they have no choice but to hide their diagnosis. Encouraging appropriate self-disclosure, with its personal and public health benefits, will thus require ongoing efforts to confront the cultural and social factors that underlie such animosity.

Still, even a more benign social climate will not make self-disclosure universal. Shame, desire, passion, fear of abandonment, lures of secrecy, vicissitudes of moral character, and qualities of relationships all mold private life and individuals' willingness to talk about HIV. Policy makers can shape the context of private choice, but the exercise of such choice remains beyond their control.

We began our study with an interest in how men and women from different backgrounds make complex decisions with profound implications for themselves and others; we closed by examining how policy makers have responded to these threats of HIV. Whatever role law, policy, and regulation may play, in the end, everyday moral norms and beliefs will be of far greater significance. Ultimately, not only the world of AIDS but our social milieu more widely will be shaped and defined by lingering moral and psychological questions. How do uninfected men and women, whether at significant risk or not, view their obligations to the sick and vulnerable? How do the infected weigh the benefits of secrecy against those of truth telling, and how do they understand moral obligations not to injure others? In a world where the escalating rates of HIV infection threaten millions of men, women, and children in Africa and Asia—regions where stigma, silence, and poverty hobble efforts at even rudimentary prevention—the complexities of the accounts presented here may provide some insights into the vast challenges that lie ahead.

In the industrialized world, these issues of medical secrecy and disclosure have begun to take on significance in contexts far removed from AIDS. Of note, diagnostic tests that uncover risks of genetic diseases are increasingly being developed, presenting individuals with difficult choices. Should I be tested? If I harbor a genetic predisposition to disease, should I tell the person with whom I want to have a child, and should we still consider having children? Should I share my secret knowledge with others at risk—my adult children, siblings, or other blood relatives? What obligations do clinicians have when faced with a patient's reluctance or refusal to disclose a blood test result that may have implications for others? What role should the law play in fostering or compelling disclosure? The encounter with AIDS in the last two decades of the twentieth century has raised intensely personal questions with broad public health significance, and the experience of those years has much to say to those who will face the genetic revolution. And all these matters take on added immediacy as the threat of terrorism has opened the way to surveillance of personal records in the name of national security.

We have raised more questions than we have answered, but illuminating the multifaceted nature of these issues has been our intent. In so doing we have been guided by the assumption that understanding these dilemmas is more crucial to their ultimate resolution than proffering simple and premature answers. While inspired by the work of such philosophers as Sissela Bok and David Nyberg, we believe that ethnographies such as this one, examining the lives of men and women affected by HIV, deepen our understanding of how moral issues get played out in everyday life, shaped by social, temporal, and spatial contexts.

Americans are at once both increasingly anxious about unwarranted intrusions on privacy and seduced by a confessional culture. In this milieu, these narratives can serve as lasting reminders of the vitality and fragility of encounters with disease, and the necessary but seemingly impossible challenges of building trust and communicating with each other in an ever uncertain world.

Code ID Number: Date:

This is a study of how people deal with their HIV test result as private, confidential information.

When did you first find out your HIV test result, and what was your reaction to it at that time?

Who was the first person you told about your HIV test result? Why did you tell that person? What was his or her reaction? How did you feel about that? Whom have you told since then? What have their reactions been? How have you felt about their reactions?

Are you in a relationship? If so, for how long?

Does this person know your HIV test result? When did you tell her or him your HIV test result? Did you wait? Why then? What did you say exactly? How did the topic come up? What was the person's reaction? How did you feel about that?

Have you ever been rejected by a potential sexual partner because of your HIV test result? What happened?

Have you had any anonymous partners / one-night stands or "pick-ups?" About how many? Did you discuss your HIV test result with any of them? How did they react? What happened? What kind of sexual activity did you engage in? Did you use condoms?

Were there any times when your HIV test result didn't come up? What happened? Did you use condoms? What kind of sexual activity did you engage in?

Were there any times when you decided not to reveal your HIV test result and said something else about your HIV test result other than the actual result? What did you say? Why did you decide not to reveal your HIV test result? How did you feel about this? Did you use condoms? What kind of sexual activity did you have with the person?

Have you had any casual partners since finding out your current HIV test result? Have you told any of them your HIV test result? Whom did you tell? Whom did you not tell? How did you decide whom to tell and what to say? Why then? How did the people react?

Who was the hardest person to tell? What made it hard for you to tell him or her?

Are there any people you thought about telling and decided not to? Why did you decide not to tell them?

Have you ever been glad about telling someone?

Have you told your parents about your HIV test result? What were the circumstances in which you told them? What was their reaction?

Have you told siblings about your HIV test result? What was their reaction?

Have there been situations in which others talked to you about what you should tell others concerning your HIV test result? Has a physician or a counselor ever spoken to you about talking to others concerning your HIV test result?

Have your feelings about telling others your HIV test result changed over time? How so?

What do you think most of your friends say about their HIV test result to sexual partners?

Do you know of anyone who has given inaccurate information about her or his HIV test result to sexual partners? Have you spoken to that person about that? What did you say? Do you think people should tell their sexual partners about their HIV test result? Why?

What do you think your sexual partners say about their HIV test result? Have you ever challenged or questioned what a sexual partner said about his or her HIV test result?

Can you tell me about any decisions you have ever had to make that involved having to tell the truth about yourself in a difficult situation?

Have you ever given inaccurate information to an anonymous partner? To a casual partner?

Has telling other people about your HIV test result ever changed the way you think about or see the result? How so?

Do you think people have looked at you at all differently because of your HIV test result? How so?

Sometimes a doctor or counselor knows that people who are HIV positive have not told their main sexual partners about the test result. What do you think a doctor or counselor should do under those circumstances?

NOTES

Introduction. Secrets, Lies, and Private Life

1. Robert Klitzman, *Being Positive: The Lives of Men and Women with HIV* (Chicago: Ivan R. Dee, 1997).

2. Erving Goffman, *The Presentation of Self in Everyday Life* (Garden City, N.Y.: Doubleday, 1959).

3. Eve Kosofsky Sedgwick, *Epistemology of the Closet* (Berkeley: University of California Press, 1990).

4. Erving Goffman, *Stigma: Notes on the Management of Spoiled Identity* (Englewood Cliffs, N.J.: Prentice-Hall, 1963).

5. Talcott Parsons, *The Social System* (Glencoe, Ill.: Free Press, 1951).

6. Clifford Geertz, *Interpretation of Culture* (New York: Basic Books, 1973).

7. Quoted in Sissela Bok, *Lying: Moral Choices in Public and Private Life* (New York: Pantheon Books, 1978), 38.

8. Sissela Bok, *Secrets: On the Ethics of Concealment and Revelation* (New York: Pantheon Books, 1982), 19.

9. David Nyberg, *The Varnished Truth: Truth Telling and Deceiving in Ordinary Life* (Chicago: University of Chicago Press, 1993), 26.

10. Thomas Nagel, "Concealment and Exposure," *Philosophy and Public Affairs* 27 (1998): 3–30.

11. Russell Hardin, *Trust and Trustworthiness* (New York: Russell Sage Foundation, 2002).

12. Tom Tyler and Roderick Kramer, "Whither Trust?" in R. Kramer and T. Tyler (eds.), *Trust in Organizations* (Thousand Oaks, Calif.: Sage, 1996).

13. Ronald Bayer, "AIDS Prevention: Sexual Ethics and Responsibility," *New England Journal of Medicine* 334 (1996): 1540–42.

14. Susan Cochran and Vickie M. Mays, "Sex, Lies, and HIV," *New England Journal of Medicine* 322 (1990): 774–75.

15. David L. Chambers, "Gay Men, AIDS and the Code of the Condom," *Harvard Civil Rights–Civil Liberties Law Review* 29 (1994): 353–85.

16. Gay Men's Health Crisis, New York, pamphlet.

17. Elisa J. Sobo, *Choosing Unsafe Sex: AIDS Risk Denial among Disadvantaged Women* (Philadelphia: University of Pennsylvania Press, 1995).

18. Jonathan Elford, Graham Bolding, Mark Maguire, et al., "Sexual Risk Behavior among Gay Men in a Relationship," *AIDS* 13 (1999): 1407-11.

19. Patricia Illingworth, *AIDS and the Good Society* (London: Routledge, 1990).

20. Michael Yeo, "Sexual Ethics and AIDS: A Liberal View," in C. Overall and W. P. Zion (eds.), *Perspectives on AIDS: Ethical and Social Issues* (Toronto: Oxford University Press, 1991), 75-90.

21. Don Des Jarlais, personal communication.

22. Institute of Medicine, *No Time to Lose: The AIDS Crisis Is Not Over* (Washington, D.C.: National Academy Press, 2000), 26.

23. U.S. House of Representatives, Committee on Commerce, *Ryan White Care Act Amendments, Report,* July 25, 2000, 32-33.

24. Robert Janssen, David Holtgrave, Ronald Valdiserri, et al., "The Serostatus Approach to Fighting the HIV Epidemic: Prevention Strategies for Infected individuals," *American Journal of Public Health* 91 (2001): 1019-24, 1023.

25. David Tuller, "New Tactic to Prevent AIDS Spread," *New York Times,* August 13, 2002, F5.

26. Jane Simoni, Hyacinth Mason, Gary Marks, et al., "Women's Self Disclosure of HIV Infection: Rates, Reasons, and Reactions," *Journal of Consulting and Clinical Psychology* 63 (1995): 474-78.

27. Robert B. Hays, Leon McKusick, and Lance Pollack, "Disclosing HIV Seropositivity to Significant Others," *AIDS* 7 (1993): 425-31, 425.

28. Ibid., 430.

29. Geertz, *Interpretation of Culture.*

30. Carol Gilligan, *In a Different Voice: Psychological Theory and Women's Development* (Cambridge: Harvard University Press, 1993).

31. Rita Charon, "The Patient-Physician Relationship. Narrative Medicine: A Model for Empathy, Reflection, Profession, and Trust," *Journal of the American Medical Association* 286 (2001): 1897-1902.

32. Anselm Strauss and Juliet Corbin, *Basics of Qualitative Research: Techniques and Procedures for Developing Grounded Theory* (Newbury Park, Calif.: Sage, 1990).

33. Concorde Coordinating Committee, "Concorde: MRC/ANRS Randomized Double-Blind Controlled Trial of Immediate and Deferred Zidovudine in Symptom-Free HIV Infection," *Lancet* 343 (1994): 8711-881.

34. Steven Deeks, Mark Smith, Mark Holodny, et al., "HIV-1 Protease Inhibitors: A Review for Clinicians," *Journal of the American Medical Association* 277 (1997): 145-53.

35. B. Carlton, "New AIDS Drugs Bring Hopes to Provincetown, but Unexpected Woes," *Wall Street Journal,* October 3, 1996, A1.

36. Robert Klitzman, Sheri Kirshenbaum, Lauren Kittell, et al., "HIV Disclosure in the Post-HAART Era," presented at *AIDS Impact: Biopsychosocial Aspects of HIV Infection,* Milan, July 7-10, 2003.

37. Susan Scheer, Priscilla Lee Chu, Jeffrey Klausner, et al., "Effect of Highly Active Antiretroviral Therapy on Diagnoses of Sexually Transmitted Diseases in People with AIDS," *Lancet* 357 (2001): 432-35.

38. David Ostrow, Kelly Fox, and Joan Chmiel, "Attitudes towards Highly Active Antiretroviral Therapy Are Associated with Sexual Risk Taking among HIV-Infected and

Uninfected Homosexual Men," *AIDS* 16 (2002): 775–79.

39. Beryl Koblin, Lucia Torian, Vince Guilin, et al., "High Prevalence of HIV Infection among Young Men Who Have Sex with Men in New York City," *AIDS* 14 (2000): 1793–1800.

40. Joseph Catania, Dennis Osmond, and Ronald Stahl, "The Continuing HIV Epidemic among Men Who Have Sex with Men," *American Journal of Public Health* 91 (2001): 907–14.

41. Ibid., 911.

42. "Cluster of HIV-Infected Adolescents and Young Adults—Mississippi, 1999," *Morbidity and Mortality Weekly Report* 49, no. 38 (2000): 861–64.

43. Susan Little, Sarah Holte, Jean-Pierre Routy, et al., "Antiretroviral Drug Resistance among Patients Recently Infected with HIV," *New England Journal of Medicine* 347 (2002): 385–94.

44. CDC, "Unrecognized HIV Infection, Risk Behaviors and Perceptions of Risk among Young Black Men Who Have Sex with Men—Six US Cities, 1994–1998," *Morbidity and Mortality Weekly Report* 51, no. 33 (2001): 733–36.

Chapter 1. Getting Tested

1. Association of State and Territorial Health Officials, *ASTHO Guide to Public Health Practice: HTLVIII Antibody Testing and Community Approaches* (Washington, D.C.: Public Health Foundation, 1985).

2. CDC, "Recommendations for Assisting in the Prevention of Perinatal Transmission of Human T-Lymphotropic Virus Type III/Lymphadenopathy-Associated Virus and Acquired Immunodeficiency Syndrome," *Morbidity and Mortality Weekly Report* (*MMWR*) 34, no. 48 (1985): 721–26, 731–32.

3. Ronald Bayer, *Private Acts, Social Consequences: AIDS and the Politics of Public Health* (New Brunswick, N.J.: Rutgers University Press, 1989), 101–15.

4. Ronald Bayer "The Dependent Center: The First Decade of the AIDS Epidemic in New York City," in David Rosner (ed.), *Hives of Sickness: Public Health and Epidemics in New York City* (New Brunswick, N.J.: Rutgers University Press, 1995).

5. Project Inform, "Doctor, Patient, and HIV: A Cooperative Relationship," *PI Perspective* 4 (1988): 3–6.

6. Jane Simoni, Penelope Demas, Hyacinth Mason, et al., "HIV Disclosure among Women of African Descent: Associations with Coping, Social Support and Psychological Adaptation," *AIDS and Behavior* 4 (2000): 147–48.

Chapter 2. Sexual Partners

1. Edward O. Laumann, John H. Gagnon, Robert T. Michael, and Stuart Michaels, *The Social Organization of Sexuality: Sexual Practices in the United States* (Chicago: University of Chicago Press, 1994), chap. 5.

2. Robert Klitzman, "MDMA (Ecstasy) Use and Its Association with High Risk Behaviors, Mental Health, and Other Factors among Gay/Bisexual Men in New York City," *Drug and Alcohol Dependence* 66 (2002): 115–25.

3. Anthony R. D'Augelli and Charlotte J. Patterson, *Lesbian, Gay, and Bisexual Identities over the Lifespan* (New York: Oxford University Press, 1995), 250.

4. Simoni, Demas, Mason, et al., "HIV Disclosure among Women of African Descent, 148.

5. Linda Niccolai, Dennis Dorst, Leann Myers, et al., "Disclosure of HIV Status to Sexual Partners: Predictors and Temporal Patterns," *Sexually Transmitted Diseases* 26 (1999): 280–85.

6. Robert Stempel, Jeffrey Moulton, and Andrew Moss, "Self-Disclosure of HIV-1 Antibody Test Results: The San Francisco General Hospital Cohort," *AIDS Education and Prevention* 7 (1995): 116–23.

7. R. Wolitski, C. Reitmeijer, and G. Goldbaum, "HIV Serostatus Disclosure among Gay and Bisexual Men in Four American Cities," *AIDS Care* 10 (1998): 599–610.

8. Gary Marks, Jean Richardson, and Norman Maldonado, "Self-Disclosure of HIV Infection to Sexual Partners," *American Journal of Public Health* 81 (1991): 1321–22.

9. Samuel Perry, Joanne Ryan, Karen Fogel, et al., "Voluntarily Informing Others of Positive HIV Test Results: Patterns of Notification by Infected Gay Men," *Hospital and Community Psychiatry* 41 (1990): 549–51.

Chapter 3. Secrets and "Secret Secrets"

1. Carl Latkin, Amy Knowlton, Valerie Forman, et al., "Injection Drug Users' Disclosure of HIV Seropositive Status to Network Members," *AIDS and Behavior* 5 (2001): 297–305.

2. Simoni, Demas, Mason, et al., "HIV Disclosure among Women of African Descent," 148.

Chapter 4. Disclosure in Other Worlds

1. American Civil Liberties Union (ACLU), *Epidemic of Fear: A Survey of AIDS Discrimination in the 1980s and Policy Recommendations for the 1990s* (New York: ACLU AIDS Project, 1990).

2. CDC, "Recommendations for Preventing Transmission of Infection with Human T-Lymphotropic Virus Type III/Lymphadenopathy-Associated Virus," *Morbidity and Mortality Weekly Report* 34, no. 45 (1985): 681–86, 691–95.

3. Lawrence Gostin, "The AIDS Litigation Project: A National Review of Government and Human Rights Commission Decisions, Page II: Discrimination," *Journal of the American Medical Association* 263 (1990): 2086–93.

4. ACLU, *Epidemic of Fear.*

5. CDC, "Recommendations for Preventing Transmission of Infection with Human T-Lymphotropic Virus Type III/Lymphadenopathy-Associated Virus during Invasive Procedures," *Morbidity and Mortality Weekly Report* 35, no. 14 (1986): 221–23.

6. Lawrence Gostin, "HIV-Infected Physicians and the Practice of Seriously Invasive Procedures," *Hastings Center Report* 19 (1989): 32–39.

7. Leonard H. Glantz, Wendy K. Mariner, and George J. Annas, "Risky Business: Setting Public Health Policy for HIV-Infected Health Care Professionals," *Milbank Quarterly* 70 (1992): 43–80.

8. *Congressional Record,* July 11, 1991, 59778.

9. Mark Carl Rom, *Fatal Extraction* (San Francisco: Jossey-Bass, 1997).

Chapter 5. Dangerous Acts

1. Edward Connor, Rhoda Sperling, R. Gelber, et al., "Reduction of Maternal-Infant Transmission of Human Immunodeficiency Virus Type 1 with Zidovudine Treatment," *New England Journal of Medicine* 331 (1994): 1173–80.

Chapter 6. Making Moral Judgments

1. *Tarasoff v. Regents of the University of California,* 551 P.2d 334 (Cal. 1976 137).

Conclusion. Secrets in Public Life

1. CDC, "Recommendations," *MMWR* 34, no. 48 (1985); *Surgeon General's Report on Acquired Immune Deficiency Syndrome* (Washington, D.C.: U.S. Public Health Service, October 1986), 33; Institute of Medicine and National Academy of Sciences, *Confronting AIDS* (Washington, D.C.: National Academy Press, 1986); *Report of the Presidential Commission on the Human Immunodeficiency Virus Epidemic* (Washington, D.C.: June 24, 1988).

2. See Ronald Bayer and Kathleen E. Toomey, "HIV Prevention and the Two Faces of Partner Notification," *American Journal of Public Health* 82 (1992): 1158–64.

3. June Osborn, "AIDS, Politics and Science," *New England Journal of Medicine* 318 (1988): 444–47.

4. Stephanie Saul, "Nassau Seeks AIDS Victims' ID's," *Newsday,* November 16, 1985, 7.

5. Ibid.

6. CDC, "Partner Notification for Preventing Human Immunodeficiency Virus (HIV) Infection—Colorado, Idaho, South Carolina, Virginia," *Morbidity and Mortality Weekly Report* 37, no. 25 (1988): 394–95.

7. J. Andrus, D. Flemming, D. Harger, et al., "Partner Notification: Can It Control Epidemic Syphilis?" *Annals of Internal Medicine* 112 (1990): 539–43.

8. Neil Schram, "Partner Notification Can Be Useful Tool against AIDS Spread," *Los Angeles Times,* June 28, 1988.

9. Bernard Dickens, "Legal Limits of AIDS Confidentiality," *Journal of the American Medical Association* 259 (1988): 3449–51.

10. Gilbert Nass, *Sexuality Today* (Boston: Jones and Bartlett, 1988), 1.

11. American Academy of Family Physicians, Board Meeting, April 18–20, 1990.

12. Isabella Wilkerson, "AMA Asks Doctors to Warn AIDS Carriers' Sex Partners," *New York Times,* July 1, 1988, A1.

13. Bayer and Toomey, "HIV Prevention," 1162.

14. James G. Hodge and Lawrence O. Gostin, "Handling Cases of Willful Exposure through HIV Partner Counseling and Referral Services," *Women's Rights Law Reporter* 23 (2001): 45–62.

15. Benjamin Neidl, "Note: The Lesser of Two Evils: New York's New HIV/AIDS Partner Notification Law and Why the Right of Privacy Must Yield to Public Health," *St Johns Law Review* 73 (1999): 1191–1238.

16. Kathleen Sullivan and Martha Field, "AIDS and the Coercive Power of the State," *Harvard Civil Rights–Civil Liberties Review* 23 (1988): 139–98.

17. Nancy Ford and Michael Quam, "AIDS Quarantine: The Legal and Practical Implications," *Journal of Legal Medicine* 8 (1987): 353–97.

18. Ronald Bayer and Amy Fairchild-Carrino, "AIDS and the Limits of Control: Public Health Orders, Quarantine, and Recalcitrant Behavior," *American Journal of Public Health* 83 (1993): 1471–76.

19. Wendy Parmet, "AIDS and Quarantine: The Revival of an Archaic Doctrine," *Hofstra Law Review* 14 (1985): 53–90.

20. Lawrence Gostin, "The Politics of AIDS: Compulsory State Powers, Public Health and Civil Liberties," *Ohio State Law Journal* 49 (1989): 1017–58.

21. Ibid.

22. Bayer and Fairchild-Carrino, "AIDS and the Limits of Control."

23. Ibid.

24. Rebecca Ruby, "Apprehending the Weapon Within: The Case for Criminalizing the Intentional Transmission of the HIV," *American Criminal Law Review* 36 (1999): 313–35.

25. American Civil Liberties Union (AIDS and Liberties Project), "Criminalizing Transmission of the Virus," ms.

26. "Alaska Governor Vetoes HIV Criminal Exposure Bill," *AIDS Policy and Law* 13 (July 24, 1998).

27. Ruby, "Apprehending the Weapon Within," 320.

28. Klitzman, *Being Positive.*

29. Goffman, *Stigma.*

30. B. DePaulo, D. Kashy, S. Kirkendol, et al., "Lying in Everyday Life," *Journal of Personality and Social Psychology* 70, no. 5 (1996): 979–95.

31. Gary Marks, Jean Richardson, and Nicole Crepaz, "Are HIV Care Providers Talking with Patients about Safer Sex and Disclosure? A Multi-Clinic Assessment," *AIDS* 16 (2002): 1953–57.

Disclosure to (*continued*)
public); in-laws, 83–85; long-term partners, 31–38, 69–70, 70–71; parents, 74–83; siblings, 85–92; wives, 32–33, 37
Discrimination. *See* Stigma
Dishonesty. *See* Lies
Drug use: disclosure and, 10, 60–61, 65, 68; sense of responsibility and, 68, 144–145; sexual behavior and, 144–145, 152, 154–155, 156–157
Duties. *See* Moral obligations

Fisher, Mary, 115

Gay men
and disclosure to: anonymous partners, 56–59; casual partners, 56–59; co-workers, 112, 114; dates, 39–40, 41, 42, 44–45, 47–48, 49; friends, 98, 104, 107, 116–118; general public, 116–118, 119–120; long-term partners, 32, 54–55, 56; parents, 74, 75–76, 78, 80–81, 81–82; siblings, 89, 90–91
and lying to: casual partners, 50; dates, 51
and secrets from: anonymous partners, 165; casual partners, 140; co-workers, 112; employers, 108–109; friends, 105–106; long-term partners, 55–56; parents, 82; siblings, 89, 90
Geertz, Clifford, 4, 12
Goffman, Erving, 2, 3, 192
Going public, 115–121
Greene, Graham, 6

Hardin, Russell, 7
Harm to others: lying and, 178–184; moral judgments of, 158–163; safer sex and, 122; unsafe sex and, 122
Harm to self. *See* Risk taking
Heterosexual men
and disclosure to: children, 94; dates, 139; former partners, 68; friends, 98, 99, 104–105; general public, 118–119; in-laws, 84; long-term partners, 52–53, 68; parents, 74, 79; sex workers,

154–155; siblings, 86; wives, 32–33, 34
and lying to long-term partners, 50, 161–163, 170–173
and secrets from: children, 92; co-workers, 111; in-laws, 83–84; long-term partners, 155–156, 168–169; parents, 82; wives, 37–38
Heterosexual women
and disclosure to: casual partners, 59–60; children, 94–95; co-workers, 112–113; dates, 40–41, 42, 43, 52; former partners, 65–66, 69–70, 71–72; friends, 97–98, 98–99, 100–101, 102, 103; general public, 115, 119, 120–121; health care workers, 26; in-laws, 84; long-term partners, 32, 33, 34, 48–49, 69–70; parents, 74, 75, 76–77, 77–78, 79–80; siblings, 85, 86–87, 88, 89
and lying to: friends, 105; long-term partners, 53
and secrets from: children, 92–93, 94; co-workers, 110–111, 111–112, 113; employers, 109; friends, 107; parents, 82–83; siblings, 90, 91
HIV, epidemiology of, 4
HIV test: benefits of, 17–18; debate over, 17–18; decisions about, 18–20; mandatory, 21–22; reactions to, 18–29
Homophobia. *See* Stigma: homosexuality and

Injecting-drug users
and disclosure to: casual partners, 65; children, 94; co-workers, 112–113, former partners, 65, 66–67; friends, 98, 99–100, 104–105; in-laws, 84; long-term partners, 43, 52–53, 68; parents, 75, 76, 79; siblings, 85, 86–87; wives, 32–33, 34, 37, 68
and lying to long-term partners, 53
and secrets from: children, 92–93; co-workers, 111, friends, 106–107; in-laws, 83–84; long-term partners, 55; parents, 82

Kant, Immanuel, 5
Kissing: disclosure and, 133; erotic gratifica-

About the Authors

Robert Klitzman, M.D., is an assistant professor of clinical psychiatry in the College of Physicians and Surgeons and the Mailman School of Public Health and is co-director of the Center for Bioethics at Columbia University. He graduated from Princeton University and Yale Medical School, completed his internship and residency at Cornell / New York Hospital, and was a Robert Wood Johnson Foundation Clinical Scholar at the University of Pennsylvania. His books include *A Year-Long Night: Tales of a Medical Internship* (1989); *In a House of Dreams and Glass: Becoming a Psychiatrist* (1995); *Being Positive: The Lives of Men and Women with HIV* (1997); and *The Trembling Mountain: A Personal Account of Kuru, Cannibals, and Mad Cow Disease* (1998), based on his field work among the Stone Age Fore group in Papua New Guinea, investigating the epidemiology and medical anthropology of the Kuru epidemic. Klitzman has written about ethical, social, and psychological issues in medicine and psychiatry for academic journals as well as for the *New York Times* and other publications. He has received several awards for his work, including a career development award from the National Institute of Mental Health, a Burroughs-Wellcome Fellowship (for future leaders in psychiatry) from the American Psychiatric Association, an Aaron Diamond Foundation Fellowship, a Picker-Commonwealth Scholar Award, a Visiting Scholar Award at the Russell Sage Foundation, and a Merck Company Foundation Fellowship at Yaddo.

Ronald Bayer, Ph.D., is a professor at the Center for the History and Ethics of Public Health, Mailman School of Public Health, Columbia University, where he has taught since 1988. Before coming to Columbia, he was at the Hastings Center, a research institute devoted to the study of ethical issues in medicine and the life sciences. Bayer's research has examined ethical and policy issues in public health, focusing especially on AIDS, tuberculosis, illicit drugs, and tobacco. His articles on AIDS have appeared in the *New England Journal of Medicine, Journal of the American Medical Association, Lancet, American Journal of Public Health,* and *Milbank Quarterly.* His books include *Homosexuality and American Psychiatry: The Politics of Diagnosis* (1981); *Private Acts, Social Consequences: AIDS and the Politics of Public Health* (1989); *AIDS in the Industrialized Democracies: Passions, Politics, and Policies* (1991, edited with David Kirp); *Blood Feuds: Blood, AIDS, and the Politics of Medical Disaster* (1999, edited with Eric Feldman); and *AIDS Doctors: Voices from the Epidemic* (2000, written with Gerald Oppenheimer). In 1995, Bayer's work was recognized by the National Institute of Mental Health when he was awarded a five-year Senior Scientist Award. In 2002 he was elected to the Institute of Medicine.